# What You Must Do to Escape the Bird Flu

Brendanne Phillips

**Warning: None of the remedies in this book have been analyzed and thoroughly tested for effectiveness by the FDA. Use them at your own risk.**

In the event of illness, this book is not meant to be a substitute for professional medical care. The information contained in this book is not a guarantee that you and your family will live through a pandemic. It is intended to help increase your chance of survival, not as a substitute for going to the doctor. Anyone who follows the information given in the following pages is doing it at their own risk.



For ordering, booking, permission, or questions, contact:

Brendanne Phillips
PO Box 10111
Titusville, FL 32783
Email orders to: bren@escapethebirdflu.com

ISBN: 0-9774513-8-0
Library of Congress Control Number: 2006939063

Cover Design: Creative Techniques

Changing Lives Publishing
www.Print2Publish

Printed in the United States of America

**In Memory of**

**Dorothy Amstadt**
**March 29, 1930 - August 12, 2002**

*"Angels fly*
*because they take*
*themselves*
*lightly"*

Gilbert K. Chesterton

# Contents

*"They did then what they knew how to do,*
*now we know better we can do better"*

Maya Angelou

# Introduction

How and why did I come to write a book on the Bird Flu? This is probably the first question that comes to your mind. It really began eleven years ago when my daughter started having ear infections. We also found out around that time, my daughter had an allergy to red dye. This was a problem because not only does penicillin have red dye, but there were a lot of other medications that contained red dye. Pain killers were out; cough syrups were no good to us. What were we to do? Every time my child had one of the products off the shelf from a drugstore, she would break out into a miserable three day long rash.

I soon learned, in order to treat the mildest of illnesses to the severe ones, we were going to have to look somewhere else for help. I finally came across a home remedy for cough syrup. It soon became my passion to find remedies we could make and use at home for my daughter.

Treating my cancer, diagnosed in 1998, using alternative therapies gave me the knowledge of how the body works. I also have run an organic food buying group for 10 years which helped me to locate alternative sources for food and supplies. I was and still am an avid reader of health information.

I started developing a plan for my family to survive the bird flu, because after surviving cancer I was not about to die of the Bird Flu. One day while watching a talk show and listening to the gentleman from the CDC, I was disappointed to learn that the only advice he was offering families was to purchase masks and stock up on food. I had spent a great deal of time before that gathering all my information and creating a plan for my family. To my surprise I had more of an idea of what to do than he did. I wrote a short pamphlet for family and friends. As I continued to research and learn, I found there was even more to learn and do for the bird flu. As I gathered more and more information the pamphlet grew into a book. I knew I had to share this information with more than just my family and friends by publishing this book.

## *What You Must do to Escape the Bird Flu*

I have decided to include folk remedies I personally use in this book. I figured if a Bird Flu does ever hit, it would be great for everyone to have some home remedies that did not involve drugs and could be made right in a person's kitchen. These same remedies can be used for the seasonal flu too!

My prayer is that there will never be a need for a book like this but I know prevention will bring peace of mind. May God be with us through these times ahead.

# 1

# What Can Happen In Just One Week

## *The Story of Sue and Tim*

At home, Sue has been reading a lot about the Bird Flu. She decided over a month ago that she should stock up on food and supplies, just in case the flu ever does arrive. She wanted to have at least two weeks of food and supplies, but her constant reading of the newspaper caused her to buy more than she had planned.

In Lebanon the Bird Flu was showing signs of mutating and being transmitted from human to human. Sue was uneasy about Tim's upcoming trip to China. She had begged Tim not to go.

Sue and Tim were living quite normal lives. Tim is an engineer for a local company and Sue is a stay at home Mother of three children: Mary, age 9; Emily, age 6; Thomas, age 2.

Tim left on Friday to oversee his company's start-up operation to build awnings and platforms for boats.

"China is far from Lebanon and besides I will be in Hong Kong on China's east coast," says Tim. He assures Sue he will be fine. "I'll be back before the Bird Flu ever reaches China."

Unbeknownst to Tim a wealthy couple and their four children had fled Lebanon just a few days before he arrived; this family became his next door neighbor in the hotel where he was staying. On several occasions, he rode up in the hotel elevator with one or more of the family members.

*The Chinese government had noticed a dramatic increase in Bird Flu cases. They also suspected that it had mutated to human to human transmission. The Chinese government was keeping this all under wraps just like they did a few years ago when Severe Acute Respiratory Syndrome (SARS) broke out. They had many diplomatic and financial relationships that could be dramatically affected if the news got out.*

## SATURDAY 11:30 P.M.
## TIM ARRIVES HOME

Despite his late night return to the United States on Saturday night, Tim is feeling well enough to go to Church on Sunday morning.

On Monday morning Tim has the sniffles, but heads off to work anyway.

## MONDAY 8:30 P.M.
## TIM FEELS SICK AND RETIRES TO BED EARLY

In the evening when he returns home he is much sicker than he was when he left that morning. He has a real bad headache, a slight fever and is coughing. He retires to bed early, attributing his illness to the recycled air on the airplane. During the night he is tossing and turning, he just can't get comfortable.

At 2:00 a.m. Sue wakes up disturbed by his constant shifting in the bed and his endless coughing fits. She turns on the light to see if there is anything she can do to make him more comfortable. As the light goes on, she sees Tim blowing his nose and notices the tissue is filled with blood. On further inspection she sees blood on the pillow and is unsure where it is coming from, until Tim turns and looks at her.

"Tim!" Sue says in a horror, "Your ear, it is all bloody!" Panic stricken, she calls one of her neighbors to come over and stay with the kids while she rushes Tim to the hospital.

## What Can Happen In Just One Week

### TUESDAY 3:00 A.M.
### TIM IS RUSHED TO THE HOSPITAL

At 3:00 a.m. they arrive at the hospital. Tim is the third case to be admitted with similar symptoms; although, his symptoms are more severe than any of the other people; the doctor tells her that it looks like Tim has the flu.

In the back of Sue's mind she fears that this could be the Bird Flu, but there were no cases reported in China. She rationalized that all of Tim's coughing and blowing of his nose must have caused the bleeding, nothing more. If it was the Bird Flu, she surely would have known it.

Sue stays at the hospital with Tim until 6:30 a.m., at which time she kisses him on the forehead and tells him after the girls are off to school; she and Thomas will be back. Thomas usually wakes up between 7:00 and 8:00 a.m.; since Thomas had never been left alone with anyone, Sue wanted to get home before he awoke to find their neighbor sleeping on the couch.

To her relief when she arrived home, Thomas was still asleep. The neighbor inquires about Tim's condition.

"The doctors say it could just be the flu," Sue replies.

"But, what about all that blood?" Says the neighbor, "You don't suppose it is the Bird Flu, do you?"

"I don't know. They say they will know more after his tests come back from the lab," says Sue.

Her neighbor gives her a look as if she had seen a ghost. "It is; I just know it!" She says, rushing to get out of the house.

After seeing her neighbor's reaction, Sue's fears get the better of her. She frantically tries to disinfect her house. She strips the bed and throws Tim's pillow and the rest of the sheets out in the trash. She is spraying cleaners and odor removers on the mattress. She is whizzing through the house, trying to remove any possible contamination; zoning in on places Tim might have touched: the phone, the toilet--the sinks, the door knobs, all are being meticulously cleaned with disinfectant. As her children arise, they find her scrubbing the kitchen floor.

Sue forgot about the children. She feels they will be safer at school while she continues to disinfect the house. Changing her mode, she stops to get the girls ready for school. The girls are out of the house by 8:30 a.m., the bus picks them up and they are on their way.

Sue opens the windows to air out the house, even though it was mid January. The bitter cold makes its way in. She only shuts the windows when she notices Thomas starting to shiver. After getting Thomas changed and fed she continues her frantic cleaning. Tim's cell phone and personal items are placed into a plastic bag and put into the garage. Part of her wants to believe that she is getting carried away worrying about nothing.

"It can't be Bird Flu," she prays, pressing on, not wanting to take any chances.

At 1:00 p.m. the school calls and says Emily is sick and should be checked out and taken home.

## TUESDAY 1:12 P.M.
## TIM DIES

Tim dies at 1:12 p.m. The nurse tries to reach Sue at home, but she is not there. The nurse leaves a message for Sue to call her at the hospital at once.

*Health officials are on the scene. Since Tim is the first to die they want to hold off telling the media until the diagnosis is confirmed. They do not want the people in the city to panic. The officials think they can contain the spread of the disease with quarantines. Since Tim was admitted, fifteen more people from his flight have been admitted to the hospital with similar symptoms.*

## TUESDAY 1:30 P.M.
## SUE ARRIVES AT SCHOOL TO PICK UP EMILY

Thirty minutes later Sue shows up at the school; the school day was just about over, so she decides to check Emily and Mary both out.

Emily is coughing, has a runny nose and a slight fever. Sue felt something was really wrong. Fearing the worst, she rushes her to the pediatrician. The pediatrician looks Emily over and counsels Sue not to worry. "It looks like just a virus," he said. Sue tells the doctor of Tim's illness and asks if he is sure it is not the Bird Flu. The doctor, having no knowledge of any reported cases of the Bird Flu in the U.S., says, "No, it is very unlikely."

Sue begs him to give her something, perhaps some Penicillin. The doctor assures her that penicillin does not work on viruses, only bacteria. Sue had to admit Emily's illness did not appear to be any worse than a normal bad cold.

"Could the doctor be right," she wondered. "Am I making more of it than I should?" After all she did not know what Tim's illness really was. Her fears were probably getting the better of her. Sue and the kids return home. Sue was quite tired; this could be why she was jumping the gun on taking Emily to the doctor. She just wasn't thinking straight.

*(A message is waiting on her answering machine, but Sue is unaware that it is there)*

Sue is too busy putting Emily to bed, giving her vitamin C and something to drink. As she is walking past the answering machine's flashing light, it goes unnoticed. Sue enters into her room and begins to flip her mattress over and make her bed. In the mean time, while Emily is resting, Mary and Thomas are playing with his train set; Sue tries to take a well needed nap.

## TUESDAY 4:00 P.M.
## EMILY IS VERY SICK

Two hours later, Sue is awaken by a scream. Mary is frantically calling out, "Emily is bleeding!! Mom, come quick!" Sue arrives at Emily's bedside to see blood running out her nose. It appeared to be no more than a normal nosebleed. This worried Sue because Emily has never had a nosebleed. Sue wasn't going to take any chances. Rushing to the phone she immediately calls the pediatrician. The office staff is bustling; five children from Emily's class had arrived in the last hour. Some had already been sent to the hospital. Sue asks the nurse on the other end of the phone, "What should I do?"

"Don't bring her back here. Take her right over to the Hospital," the nurse instructed.

Sue had no extended family in town. She could not ask a friend for help at the risk of exposing their children. She knew calling her neighbor was out. Should she leave her nine year old home alone with two year old Thomas? Where would they be safer? Was it better to bring them with her, because her house was already contaminated? What to do? As Sue saw it, she had no choice, but to take all the kids to the hospital with her.

## TUESDAY 4:15 P.M.
## A QUARANTINE IS IMPOSED AND SUE IS STOPPED FROM TAKING EMILY TO THE HOSPITAL

As she is packing the kids up in the van, an armed truck pulls up and blocks her driveway. Several military men carrying guns rush from the truck. One calls out, "Get back in the house, Ma'am! This house is being quarantined by orders of the U.S. government!"

"It can't be. I need to get this child to the hospital, Now!" Sue says, as panic gripped her.

"A medical team will be arriving shortly to assess the situation."

A frightened Sue asks-- not wanting to know-- but the scene being played out told her it was true-- "It's Bird Flu, isn't it?"

"Yes, Ma'am and we don't want it to spread any further." The men continued to have their guns drawn.

Sue had no choice but to take the kids inside. She tries to call the pediatrician again, but to no avail, the line is busy.

Emily was crying "My bones hurt, mommy." Sue tilted her head back, pinching her nose, to stop the bleeding, trying to make her comfortable. Her fever had climbed to 104.3. Sue was giving her medication to reduce the fever, aches and pains, along with cough suppressants to suppress her cough. Emily is vomiting into a bowl. Mucus is coming up when she vomits. She says, "I can't breathe." Emily is getting sicker by the moment.

*(The flashing light on the answering machine still goes unnoticed)*

"Where is that medical team? Why aren't they here?" Sue is emotional as she is frantically trying to care for her daughter. The day becomes night. No medical team arrives. Mary is doing a wonderful job taking care of Thomas. Sue only had to step in when Thomas had a real messy diaper. Sue moved Mary's mattress from Emily and Mary's room to the floor in Thomas's room, so Emily's constant coughing would not keep Mary up. It was a rough night. Sue is trying to help her daughter, by making her as comfortable as possible. Another night passes where Sue gets very little sleep.

## WEDNESDAY MORNING 5:00 A.M.
## SUE LEARNS TIM DIED

At 5:00 a.m. Sue goes to her room to change, throws cold water on her face and walks down the hall to see the answering machine light flashing, signaling a message. She stops to listen to the message. It is an urgent message from the hospital.

"Oh my God!" she says. As she dials the hospital she says, "Please, God, let him be okay!" In her panic and stress to take care of her sick daughter and the other children, she had not had the time to check on Tim. The hospital staff answers.

"I am checking on a patient named Tim Smith. Can you tell me how he is doing?"

"Ma'am, we don't have time for this. The hospital is packed with people needing service. You will have to come in to check on him," responded the lady on the other end of the phone.

"But, I was given this number saying there was an urgent message regarding Tim---"

The lady interrupted Sue, "Then, let me check on that for you. You said his name is Tim Smith?"

"Yes, that's right," said Sue.

The lady comes back to the phone. "Is this Mrs. Smith?"

"Yes"

"The call was to notify you that at 1:15 p.m. we are sorry to say, Tim passed away."

"No, there must be some mistake!!" said Sue.

"Ma'am, we have had a number of people who have died today. It was confirmed that he died of the Bird Flu. The government has been notified and you should have been quarantined by now."

Sue's worst fears had been confirmed. She knew Tim had the Bird Flu but she kept on praying that he some how would make it through. After all he was in the hospital.

*By this time Wednesday morning the news is saying that an out break of the Bird Flu exists; however, all those that may have been exposed have been put under a guarded strict quarantine. The rest of the population should not worry. Everything is under control. People are worrying, panicking anyway. They are hitting the markets, snatching up all the food they can. Fights are breaking out in the grocery stores. Some people are being gluttons, trying to take everything they can and not sharing what is there.*

Sue now must keep her attention on Emily. Emily is getting blue patches on her skin. Sue does not realize this is a sign that Emily is not getting enough oxygen into her system. Her lungs are filling up with fluid as she gasps for air. Sue is at her bedside, crying, wanting to help but not knowing what to do.

## WEDNESDAY 7:00 A.M.
## EMILY DIES

At 7:00 a.m. Emily gasps her last breath of air. She is gone. Mary and Thomas are not awake yet. Sue is emotionally beaten, tears run down her face. In a matter of days she has lost both a husband and a child.

A knock comes at the door. Sue opens the door to find men dressed in white from head to toe. It was the medical team. They are too late to make a difference, too late to help Emily. They are holding a big "quarantined" sign.

"Ma'am, we need to put this on your door," one of the guardsmen instructed.

"You are not to come outside for any reason; the National Guard posted outside has orders to shoot, if you choose to do otherwise."

As if Sue's losses weren't enough, hearing the demands of these men, she is at a loss for words, but finally says, "What if I need something like medical attention or food?"

"We'll worry about that when the time comes," said one of the guardsmen.

"Well, you are too late, my daughter passed away less than an hour ago!" Shaken by the memories, she begins to sob.

The men in white clothes continue, "Is she your only child?"

"No, I have two others."

"We must get her out immediately, so as not to further expose the others?" The man said with authority. The men leave for a moment and return to the house with a body bag in hand. They enter the home and remove the child from her bed and place her into the bag.

"Where are you taking her?" Sue questioned.

"All bodies are being taken to a county morgue for evaluation."

Sue could not bear the fact that her little child was reduced to being called a body. She was no longer a person but a body. To them she was something that needed to be examined and disposed of, not loved and cherished. Sue knew she had to let them take her. Thank God Mary and Thomas slept through the whole ordeal. Sue knew that when they awoke she would not be able to bear to tell them that both their father and Emily had died. After Emily's body was taken out Sue went to work cleaning up the room. She stops as soon as she hears a door open. Thomas is up. The men in white had left just in time. She locks Emily's room as she is coming out. Mary is right behind Thomas.

"Mom, is Emily okay?" Mary inquires.

"She is sleeping. We need to let her sleep as much as possible. I don't want anyone going into this room. Okay?"

"Are you okay, Mom?"

Sue is not about to tell a nine year old that her father and sister have passed away. "I'm really tired and need to get some sleep."

"I'll watch Thomas if you want to take a nap," said Mary.

Sue changes Thomas's diaper and prepares breakfast for the two of them before heading off for a nap. Sue, so emotionally exhausted and lacking in sleep, says, "Mary, I'm going to go take a nap now. If anyone comes to the door, do not open it; come and get me, okay?"

"Okay, but for how long?"

"I don't know. If I'm not up in a couple of hours, wake me up."

Mary and Thomas watch a DVD while their mother gets some much needed sleep.

*The news is reporting more cases are being admitted to the local hospital, but not to worry hospitals are stepping up to the plate and containing the problem. Quarantines are being placed on all those that have been in direct contact with the ill.*

## WEDNESDAY EVENING
## SUE IS BECOMING ILL

After what Sue thought was only a few hours of sleep, she awakes to find it is dark outside. She jumps out of bed and runs out into the living room, not sure of what she will find.

Mary is playing cards with Thomas. "Oh, you're awake, Mom."

At first Sue thinks it has all been a nightmare until Mary continues: "Emily hasn't been coughing. Should I go in and wake her up?"

"No!" Sue blurts out, trying to cover her tracks: "The best thing for a sick person is sleep. You must not go in and wake her up. Promise me you won't."

"Okay, I was just trying to help. I got Thomas and me some lunch and something for dinner. I changed his diaper three times all by myself" Mary proudly proclaimed.

"I'm so proud of you, Mary." Sue hugs and holds her as she silently cries.

Sue notices the kitchen is a mess and starts to clean it up. The next morning Sue is coughing and not feeling well. Thomas has a runny nose. Mary is fine. By nightfall, Sue has aches and pains and a fever. She is popping Vitamin C like crazy and giving her children the same, taking way more than the daily recommended allowance.

## THURSDAY MORNING
## SUE TRIES TO GO TO THE HOSPITAL, BUT IS STOPPED BY THE GUARDSMEN

Sue is feeling sicker and sicker. She tries to get help by going to the men at the end of the driveway.

"Ma'am, don't come any closer! Get back in the house! I am instructed to shoot if you try to leave," said the guardsmen.

"But, I need help! I need medical attention! I have two small children! Please help me!"

"Get back in the house NOW! Or I'll have to shoot! Don't make me do it!"

Getting shot wouldn't help the kids. As she turns to go back in the house, she calls out, "If you care at all, get the medical team back here as soon as possible!"

Sue is shocked. Now she is afraid of touching her own children. Remembering that she had some supplies, Sue begins to give Mary instructions on what to do if she gets sicker. Sue writes notes and places them where Mary will find them. She fears she does not have enough supplies since she does not know how long the quarantine will last. Thursday night her health begins to wane, her fever is 106.2, she is having trouble thinking. The next morning she calls out for Tim. Sue has become delirious and incoherent. Mary comes rushing in to give her mother some water and Vitamin C.

Nine year old Mary is now in charge of the household. Frantic, she tries to get help from the men outside, but, like her mother, they ordered her back inside. The little girl's pleas for help are ignored.

*The news is finally admitting there is a problem. The hospitals are full and have no more room. The quarantines are not working. 29 people died on Tuesday, 67 on Wednesday and 139 on Thursday. The count is going up rather fast. People are refusing to go to work; the grocery stores are not being stocked because truck drivers are refusing to enter the city. Five more cities are under siege. The Bird Flu is spreading fast with quarantines showing little, if any, signs of having any affect on the spreading of the disease.*

This Scenario is a fictional account of how quickly things can progress when the Bird Flu develops into human-to-human transmission. This story was developed from many accounts of similar events that happened during the flu of 1918. If the Bird Flu were to return today similar events could happen again.

*"One should ......be able to*
*see things as hopeless*
*and yet be determined*
*to make them otherwise"*

F. Scott Fitzgerald

# 2

# Bird Flu: It's Coming!

## *Are you ready?*

No longer will money secure our future. If money becomes invalid, we will still require food, water and the knowledge in how to survive. Storing grains without knowing how to cook them is like having a well for water, with no electricity to get it to the surface, pointless.

Only 10% of the women in the U.S. know how to cook from a recipe and only 1% know how to process grains into edible food. A lot of talents have given way to progress: farming, gardening, hunting, sewing and cooking. These are vital survival skills. If our world suffers a global disaster the people with the knowledge of these skills will survive. We should take the time to learn these skills to ensure our survival of the Bird Flu or other crisis.

Why be ready? We live in complicated times. Many disasters threaten our world today: terrorist attacks, global warming, over population, and natural disasters, like hurricanes, earthquakes, and floods. It is just a matter of time before one of these disasters directly affects our lives. Which one will it be? How will our lives fit into the mix? Who will have the power? What will be the currency?

Great civilizations have fallen into extinction before: such as the Mayan, the Roman and many others. We should not be so arrogant as to believe that it can not happen today. The Bird Flu is coming! Are you ready? We need to listen to the warnings of the

Center for Disease Control (CDC) and take them seriously. If the experts say it is coming why not "*Err on the side of caution*" and heed their warning? If we choose not to prepare and Bird Flu does arrive the disaster could bring down our country. If we do prepare and in the slim chance Bird Flu does not develop we can use our resources on smaller disasters like earthquakes, hurricanes, snowstorms and floods. The only thing that makes sense is to prepare. We must prepare our country, because when people are prepared, they are not afraid. We saw with Hurricane Katrina what happens when people are afraid. People in the Super Dome felt there was little hope, and they reacted out of fear with dire consequences. If people are hopeful they will help their neighbor. When they feel lost and forgotten their fear will overwhelm them.

## WHEN FEAR OVERWHELMS

- **Morals deteriorate**
- **People fight for survival**
- **People fight for resources**
- **People die needlessly**

To wait and hope that the Bird Flu is all an unnecessary scare is like refusing to leave when a category five hurricane is heading your way, and hoping that it may turn and you will be saved. Hoping you will not die is not a solution. Preparing for the worst and hoping for the best is. Don't you think those who were left in the Super Dome, in hindsight, would rather have spent two days walking out of harms way, rather than suffering in the Super Dome disaster. You are there NOW, and you are being warned that a storm is coming, the Bird Flu. Are you going to be ready for it, or find yourself among those lost in the storm?

# 3

# What Is The Bird Flu?

## *Where does it come from?*

In 1997 the Bird Flu appeared in Hong Kong, China among poultry workers who had direct contact with infected birds. Until five people died from the Bird Flu in the summer of 2006, the only people who died from the Bird Flu were those that had direct contact with the ill birds. It was believed that not all those who died, in 2006, had direct contact with birds. This confused the officials. Had the Bird Flu become now human to human transmittable? At first the indication seemed that it very likely could have; however, after the experts examined the viruses genetic code it still shows no signs that it has mutated to human to human transmission. Even though it may not be human to human transmittable, the disease is showing signs of becoming more aggressive.

In history the Bird Flu's have taken on many names, such as Spanish Flu, Avian Flu, Pandemic of 1918, Hong Kong Flu, H5N1 virus and Swine Flu. These are not all the exactly genetically identical flu but they are all flu's that originated in birds. Even the yearly less severe seasonal flu viruses have their origin in birds, according to John M. Barry, *The Great Influenza*, pg. 451.

*"It is our attitude*
*towards events*
*not events themselves,*
*which we can control."*

Epictetus

# 4

# How Does It Spread?

## *How will it affect my family?*

The first thing you need to understand is the problem itself. What the Bird Flu is and how it can affect you. Then, you will be ready to do something about preparing for it. Bird Flu starts out simply in one area, and then it spreads.

Do you remember the hair commercial some time back, where you try the hair product and then tell two friends and then they tell two friends and so forth? That commercial is a great example of just how rapidly a Bird Flu can spread. This is what happens with Bird Flu; it begins and then starts to spread. As it spreads, it begins slowly, and then advances more and more rapidly, like wild fire. Soon, it is out of control. This happens because, unlike wild fire, it is harder to see Bird Flu coming. Also, authorities will believe they can contain it.

We cannot rely on quarantines to halt the spread of the disease. Bird Flu will refuse to be contained. We will not be able to kill enough birds, or isolate enough cases to stop it. In 1918 towns that isolated themselves still had the disease get past their defenses. This most likely happens, because it is difficult to prevent wild birds and other animals from penetrating the borders.

We can see Bird Flu coming, unlike in 1918. Today we have migratory maps showing its progress. Where the migratory routes overlap, the disease spreads among the bird population. Migrating birds get the Bird Flu and then migrate to different areas as the seasons change.

As the Bird Flu moves along migratory routes, we see the spread of deaths in the human populations are following these same migratory routes. We can monitor countries a half world away.

As the Bird Flu spreads across the world, more and more people are getting the flu directly from the birds. Even other mammals are showing up with the disease. A cat in Germany is believed to have gotten the illness directly from a bird. This is of great concern, because if more mammals are getting the illness, this will allow for it to easily mutate, or the viruses to mix. We know it is just a matter of time before it mutates. The way a virus mutates or mixes is by a human or animal contracting two viruses at the same time; the viruses exchange proteins and create a new super virus. As more people and mammals become infected with the original Bird Flu disease, the chances of mutation, or a mixing of illnesses, become greater and greater. The possibility of producing a super flu is heightened. More cases of Bird Flu will increase the chance the virus will have an opportunity to mutate into a super virus.

How do Bird Flu's and pandemics develop? Many do not realize that the catastrophic flu of 1918 was a Bird Flu. A Bird Flu developed into a pandemic once and it can do it again. Since most humans cannot get bird diseases (H5N1), and most birds cannot get human diseases, how does a Bird Flu become a human flu pandemic? We know it does occur, as shown in 1918. Occasionally, a bird disease makes that species jump, allowing humans to acquire it. Experts agree that today's bird disease, which began in 1997, in its current form does not yet have the capability to be transmitted from human to human. It must be obtained from direct contact with birds.

In 1900 a Bird Flu existed like the 1997 Bird Flu. It took 18 years to develop into a deadly virus. If we are following the same timeline, 2007 would be year ten, this gives us only eight more years to prepare, or does it? We cannot count on having that much time, because there are indicators that it might develop sooner

Today the influenza viruses are getting more virulent (becoming more deadly). This is one indicator that we need to prepare now. But, eight years is a long time. What made the 1918 flu so deadly was the stress of WWI. All we need is a stressful event mixed with a record cold winter, which will give the virus the opportunity to mutate into a deadly pandemic. It can happen that quickly, and since we cannot guarantee a terrorist attack, natural disaster or a record cold winter will not occur; we need to be ready NOW!

What if the London authorities, in the fall of 2006, had not caught those plotting to blow up a number of commercial airliners? The fear and stress could have allowed the virus to develop into a deadly strain that winter. The fear and panic from the terrorist attacks could have translated into stress on many people's immune systems, resulting in an increased number of seasonal flu cases that winter. The more people around the world getting the seasonal flu, the higher the chance a mixing of flu's can occur, resulting in a Bird Flu mutation causing a pandemic.

Will today's Bird Flu become the 1918 flu with high death rates? Will it be another false scare like the swine flu of 1976? It is possible that a pandemic like the 1918 flu can happen. At one point, the disease in 1918 was killing an alarming 7-10% of the population. 10% does not seem like that much, but when we think about the figures and put them in perspective, it shows an overwhelming amount of deaths.

For example, a small city with a population of 40,000 could have a death toll near 4,000 in a matter of a year and a half. Another illustration of the magnitude of deaths that could occur: if you live on a street that has 40 houses with approximately four people per house, the deaths on your street alone could reach 16+ in 18 months. This is quite a staggering amount. This is the enormous scale of what I am talking about. A lot of people can die if the pandemic of 1918 were to repeat itself. Some people are saying this could not happen today, because things are a lot different now. Yes, many things are different now, but are they better? Are we less stressed? Is our modern life style healthier or leaving us more vulnerable?

In 1918 the most deaths were in the winter months and seemed to correlate to when a city's first outbreak occurred. Philadelphia had its first case before San Francisco. Philadelphia lost most of their flu victims in October while San Francisco's highest casualties were in the month of November. The outbreaks of the flu began in port cities. These cities were hubs for the main transoceanic transportation during that time. This is where people and goods from overseas entered the U.S. Today, since international airports, as well as seaports, are our transportation thresholds, we could have a much larger problem. Our use of air transportation increases the number of entry points into our country, making us more vulnerable. A pandemic would most likely show up in and around international air and sea ports. More points of entry could mean more widespread disease. Does this sound like we are better off, than in 1918? The world is now much smaller.

There are many medical advances that have been made in the past century, that were not available in 1918. Medicine has come a long way; we have penicillin, Tamiflu and other options, which may aid in recovery. However, will they be available? Penicillin may help once a bacterial infection is developed, but half of those who died in 1918 did not have a bacterial infection. The bacterial infection in 1918 was Pfeiffer's bacillus which has been known to be antibiotic resistant. So, if the bacteria associated with the new flu is penicillin resistant, then what? Also, will there be enough Tamiflu to go around and will it even work? After all, Tamiflu does not cure anyone of the flu, it only decreases the number of days you are sick.

Viruses are known to mutate at an alarming rate. In just hours viruses can mutate rendering medications that once worked useless. Again, does this sound like we are better off? Is our modern life style healthier? Daily we are being reminded through books, the press and other media that our stressful lives have left us with bodies that are stressed out, obese, malnourished or do not get enough exercise.

## STRESSFUL LIVES HAVE LEFT US

- **Stressed out**
- **Obese**
- **Over worked**
- **Malnourished**
- **Under Exercised**

Will our modern diet and life style cause us to have weaker immune systems? Only time will tell. Being prepared will not hurt you. Thinking you don't need to prepare can have devastating consequences.

*"Faced with crisis,*
*the man of character*
*falls back on himself."*

Charles De Gaulle

# 5

# What Will It Look Like?

## *How will I know what the Bird Flu looks like?*

What will the Bird Flu look like? In a matter of days many will become ill, fifty percent of the population could all be ill at one time. People will be afraid to go into work. Doctors and nurses may also be ill. Hospitals will be turning away people at the door. People that did not heed the warning will be panicking and have no idea what to do.

The illness will begin like a normal flu. There is no way to see it coming. Like in 1918, officials will think it is just another influenza that appears in the winter, like any other year. They will think there is nothing to fear but it should be taken seriously. Those that fall ill will have headaches, body aches, fevers, sore throats and coughing. In a matter of hours, the aches will become more and more intense, the coughing even more labored. In a few more hours blood could start pouring out of the victim's nose, ears and eye sockets. When the ill person's lungs cannot take in adequate oxygen their body will start to show signs of oxygen deprivation. This lack of oxygen will cause the victim's skin to begin to turn blue, starting with patches and soon covering the entire surface of the skin. Breathing will become more and more difficult. The ill person will panic as they frantically gasp for air.

After a person finally develops signs of being ill, it is likely that within 24 hours the first person could die. The government and health officials will still not recognize the pandemic is beginning, still insisting it is just going to be a bad flu year. The amount of deaths will have to exceed the normal expected deaths before a pandemic is realized. A few will die the first day, then double or triple the next, and within a week there will be an overload of deaths every day, exceeding 250 per week. Before you know it, hospitals will be closing their doors, because they will be filled to capacity and understaffed. The pandemic will spread like wild fire, taking everyone by surprise. Cities and towns will have no time to prepare. Panic will spread quickly. People will be in fear. Bodies will pile up, because there is no one to take them away, and no place to put them. Nurses doing in-home services will be held hostage.

Your loved one that did make it to the hospital will lie in agony. The doctor or nurse on call may have taken ill. You will not be able to go in and see your loved one, because you are at home nursing another relative that has become ill. In 1918 it was not uncommon for there to be three deaths in a single family. When you do finally make it to the hospital, you find your loved one has passed away and you are unable to claim the body. Because of the confusion in the hospital your loved one's body cannot be located; the staff is overwhelmed, caring for the living and dying. Dead people are not a top priority. Funeral home capacities are stretched to the limits, they have no more coffins. The state or County Coroners Office should be taking over for the funeral homes in an emergency, but they are overwhelmed because so many are dying. You go home in distress over the disease and soon are ill yourself; however, you have children and you must take care of them. Your oldest daughter, age 9, is now trying to take care of you and her younger brother and sister. No one is left to help! Your neighbors and friends are all going through the same thing.

An over exaggeration you say? This is exactly what happened in 1918. This alone should provoke you to being prepared. If you cannot get your spouse or children to do what is necessary, do it yourself. Be the rock in the time of distress.

# 6

# It Is All Up To You

## *Your best chance of survival is in your hands!*

You've been hearing more in the news about the potential arrival of the Bird Flu. You have resigned yourself to the fact that it is coming. Now you want to be prepared. If you are feeling confused and hopeless, after reading this book you will have the information you need to give you hope that you and your family will have the best chance of surviving a pandemic.

Is the Bird Flu a Hoax? I think not! If you were to ask Colonel Charles Hagadorn and the director of Philadelphia Department of Public Health, Dr. Wilmer Krusen, they would surely say today, "*Better safe than sorry*." Both of these men refused to heed the warning of an impending pandemic in 1918.

Colonel Hagadorn was a well respected decorated commander. It was under his command at Camp Grant, in Illinois, where during the 1918 pandemic over 500 men lost their lives in a matter of weeks. Colonel Hagadorn refused to heed the warning by the health officials. He decided to go against their advice by over loading the barracks with troops. On September 21st the first man took ill; by October 8 the devastation was enormous. Hagadorn was taken totally by surprise. Distraught by his own refusal to heed the warning, he took his own life, committing suicide by gun shot on October 8th. To him the pandemic was no hoax.

Colonel Hagadorn refused to accept the warning, will you? Dr. Wilmer Krusen denied the presence of influenza, right before a parade in Philadelphia, insisting that the city was not under any threat; therefore, he allowed the Liberty Loan Parade to go on as scheduled. In a matter of 72 hours after the parade, many of the hospitals were so over loaded with cases that they had to close their doors.

No one can say for sure if a pandemic will or will not hit or when, but being prepared is the only thing that makes sense. We write wills to prepare for our death. We have insurance, just in case we become ill, or have an accident. We wear our seatbelts in our cars in case we are ever in a collision. We prepare our homes for hurricanes or other severe weather. So, why wouldn't we want to prepare for the Bird Flu?

At this point in time, the Bird Flu virus is not transmittable from human to human, but humans can acquire the illness if they are in direct contact with birds or bird excrements. The opinion of the scientific and medical community today is that the current Bird Flu will become like the flu of 1918 and be just as deadly.

The Bird Flu of 1918 is our greatest example of what we could be facing if a pandemic were to develop today. I will be referring to Alfred Crosby's book *Epidemic and Peace, 1918.* Alfred Crosby is a researcher and authority on the 1918 flu pandemic.

John Barry's book, *The Great Influenza* is an even more detailed account of the flu of 1918. His book is a long, but excellent book on the history of medicine and how it played a role in the pandemic of 1918. It, being more current, took Crosby's book one-step further. (See Appendix A for more information).

Much can be learned from studying the pandemic of 1918, and can be applied to today's Bird Flu.

# 7

# Controlling Stress Is Key To Survival

***They say there is nothing you can do to prepare. IT IS NOT TRUE!***

In order for you to best understand what you can do to defend yourself against the Bird Flu, you must first understand a pandemic itself, its characteristics, potential to do harm, how and when a flu could appear, what causes it, and who is most susceptible to the disease. Once armed with this knowledge, then you will understand how the protocol required to protect your life will work.

To illustrate this point, think of a person who is ill and told they need to drink a lot of fluids. If the ill person doesn't bother to try to understand the reason for drinking water they could put their own life in danger. If they don't realize that some liquids, such as coffee, act as diuretics, they could end up drinking the wrong fluids. (Diuretics cause an increased amount of fluids in the body to be lost through the urine.) Since the ill person has a lack of understanding about the whole purpose of drinking water they assume any liquid will do. Then they rationalize that drinking coffee instead of water is good, because it is a fluid and they like it better. This lack of understanding could put an ill person's health in jeopardy because they didn't understand that water is needed to hydrate the body. I want to make sure that a misunderstanding of the Bird Flu doesn't happen to you.

Your understanding of the how's and why's of the 1918 flu will give you the best knowledge needed to survive the Bird Flu. The experts have tried to warn and give us advice. Their advice to protect our family is to have masks ready to wear, and to stock up on food and supplies. A lot of information exists that will further allow us to prepare our lives for a pandemic. The biggest misfortune about the 1918 flu was not being able to see the impending doom of the Bird Flu; therefore, not being able to prepare. We have the opportunity to see it coming. We can take action now!

## CONTROLLING STRESS IS KEY TO SURVIVAL

During a Bird Flu pandemic there is bound to be a lot of fear. This fear will come in the form of outside and inside stresses being put on the body.

### OUTSIDE THE BODY STRESSES

- **Overworking**
- **Smog**
- **Smoking**
- **Drinking alcohol**
- **Eating poorly**

As the threat gets closer, people will be overworking. They will feel a need to work more so that they can have extra money to put into stocking up on supplies or to put away in case they cannot work for a while due to illness, or out of the fear of leaving their home. Their worries may lead to smoking, eating or drinking more.

## INSIDE THE BODY STRESSES

- **Worries**
- **Grief**
- **Fatigue**
- **Loss of sleep**
- **Fear**

The emotional worries that come with the possible threat of a Bird Flu will result in internal stresses being placed on the body. As the threat of an impending pandemic draws closer, people will have trouble sleeping, because their fears are keeping them up at night. They will worry about the overcrowded medical facilities, that a family member may get sick and whether there is enough time to prepare. All of these negative thoughts will cause a person to develop stress.

We need to learn how to deal with our stress NOW before the Bird Flu hits. This will give us a plan or way for us to deal with our stress. Waiting to figure out how to deal with stress during a pandemic will leave you without the tools needed to manage your stress properly. Stress reduction tools are meditation, breathing technique tapes or CDs, supplements that calm nerves, or exercising equipment. We should all have a plan and know what works for us before we need to address the situation.

The first step in preparing to deal with stress is to recognize managing stress will be a problem. Knowing stress will play a major role in who gets sick and who doesn't, will give us power over the disease process. Stress is a very important factor when discussing any illness. Why is stress so important? Think about past stressful events in your life, how did you respond to stress? Did you get angry, have trouble sleeping, lose your appetite or make poor eating choices to ease the pain? Did you feel the need to exert yourself physically or push yourself past your limits? We all have experienced the negative effects of stress in our lives. There is a reason for the old adage saying *"Stress Kills,"* because it does! Ask any doctor about the effects of stress on the body and you will hear the same. What have the experts said about stress?

*"... when the tension and anxiety of modern life keeps the stress response 'on' continually, the hormones lower our resistance to disease..."*

Bernie Siegel M.D.

*"If you want to decrease the impact of stress in your life, which may result in lower cortisol levels, be sure to get regular exercise and sufficient sleep. Incorporate meditation and relaxation techniques into your daily routine."*

Andrew Weil M.D.

If you want to understand in depth how stress affects disease, further technical information can be found in Appendix A.

When dealing with any illness you must first ask yourself: *"How did I get this illness?"* Then, ask yourself, *"Was getting the illness due to a stress of any kind?"* Finally, *"Was I exposed to the illness?"*

## HOW DID I GET THIS ILLNESS?

### 1) Am I over-stressed?

**a) Did I overwork?**
**( physical stress )**

**b) Have I recently experienced an emotional event?**
**( mental stress )**

**c) Did I eat poorly, smoke, or drink alcohol?**
**( chemical stress )**

**d) Did I get enough sleep?**
**( sleep deprived stress )**

### 2) Have I been around anyone who has been sick?

By answering "yes," to any of the above questions you are at risk of becoming ill, because your body chemistry is very virus friendly and you have been exposed to an illness. A virus friendly body is one where viruses can easily grow and multiply in the body. In simple terms, the amount of stress and what kind of stress you are under will affect your health.

The biggest misconception of health is when people make the assumption that the physically fit are healthy. A physically fit body does in no way mean that the person is healthy. We have heard many times in the news about an athlete that was in prime physical shape who passed away from a heart attack or other ailment. They were physically fit but obviously not healthy; dropping dead without warning. Could their bodies on the inside have been stressed, causing a failure in their systems? Did the athlete have high cholesterol or weak veins due to an unhealthy lifestyle? Having a strong physically appearing body is a good start but not the complete answer to health.

Mr. Olf, from 1918 (whom I will discuss in great detail later), was known for his great strength but was he healthy? Mr. Olf in Crosby's book was described as a healthy person and an example of how young and healthy people died prematurely. Mr. Olf was not only known for his strength, but also for drinking 25 Martinis' at one sitting-- not a healthy thing to do, since alcohol depletes the body of vitamin C and stresses the liver. He was strong but remember over exercising (physically) can put undue stress on the body. Could he have been over exercising? A healthy body is not necessarily a body that has been stressed physically and has a lot of muscles, but a body that has been fed nutrient dense food, obtains plenty of rest and moderate exercise, and is not under any mental stress. The answer to the question is Mr. Olf was probably strong; however, he was not healthy.

## A HEALTHY BODY

- **Is not over stressed**
- **Obtains plenty of rest**
- **Obtains moderate exercise**
- **Is fed nutrient dense foods**

What is stress and how does one get stressed? The body can be stressed by one or a combination of four individual *Stress Factors*:

## STRESS FACTORS

- **Physical stress**
- **Mental stress**
- **Chemical stress**
- **Sleep deprived stress**

Physical stress is strain put on the body through physical means. A physical stress could be a sudden change in temperature; someone over working physically or over exercising the body. Pushing a body physically will put a strain on the body by causing it to use its resources to perform rather than strengthen its immune system, leaving the immune system unprepared to fight disease.

Mental stress is tension that is often not seen and often emotional. It is caused by - someone losing a job, experiencing a death of a love one, caring for a sick relative, or heading off to war. Mental stresses are usually associated with tension caused by extreme emotion.

Chemical stress is a strain put on the body by not eating nutritionally dense foods. A chemical stress on the body is eating sugar, nutritionally deprived foods, or doing something like drinking alcohol or smoking. It is a chemical reaction that takes place in the body, throwing off its natural chemical balance, causing the body to compensate for the chemical change. For example, drinking too much water can cause an electrolyte imbalance. Alcohol dehydrates the body, causing a lack of water in the body. Our body needs to stay in chemical balance in order to stay healthy.

Sleep deprived stress is caused by not getting the needed rest the body requires to maintain health, staying up late, being unable to get to sleep or being awakened in the middle of the night. Sleep deprived stress is often caused by worries and frustrations.

An example of a person with combination stress is someone that has just had a baby. If you are the mother, the combined stresses put on your body are: physical stress - from giving birth; mental stress - new parental responsibilities; and sleep deprivation stress - since most newborns do not sleep through the night for the first four months. There are a number of different stress combinations that can dramatically affect your immune system.

Combating stress is a key factor in preventing illness. Dr. Bernie Siegel in his audiotape *Laughter is the Best Medicine* and his book, *Love, Medicine & Miracles*, points out how a positive environment can influence disease. One thing he recommends is checking out any video you find funny from the library and watching it to make you laugh. Bernie Siegel has been a pioneer in the field of cancer treatment and the mind-body effects. He found that laughing will have a positive effect on the body and can increase an ill person's chance of survival.

Stress placed on your body will make it easier for a virus to take hold. The chemistry of your body will determine whether or not you can develop an illness. You will need to learn how to deal with stress in order to survive. Meditation, slow breathing and prayer will help your body cope with the stresses of life. Marianne Williamson has a great *Morning and Evening Meditation* audio. I found her audio most helpful when I was going through my cancer treatment. Dr. Andrew Weil has a CD out called, *Breathing, the Master Key to Self Healing*. The breathing exercises are designed to help the body increase lung capacity and also ease stress. Exercising will reduce your stress by addressing the sometimes negative affects of our fight or flight mechanism. I will go into this in greater detail later.

## COMBATING STRESS

- **Get plenty of rest**
- **Watch funny shows**
- **Meditate and pray regularly**
- **Do Breathing exercises**
- **Physically Exercise**

Taking an active role now will help you to be prepared for the Bird Flu. Don't wait! There will not be time to try to learn these techniques during a pandemic. Get started now!

# 8

# What Did We Learn From The 1918 Bird Flu?

## *Your grandparents survived and so can you*

Reducing stress is not the only thing you can do to prepare for the Bird Flu. Understanding why your grandparents survived gives us more clues in how we can survive, too. Your grandparents or great grandparents obviously survived the flu of 1918, or you would not be here. How and why did they survive? Were they in parts of the country less affected? Did they live in a way that increased their chances of surviving?

Historians and Scientists all agree that a Bird Flu was responsible for the 1918 flu epidemic. Where the illness began has been a big debate. Did it start in the U.S., China or come from France? It doesn't matter how it got here, only that it did. It is theorized that the 1918 flu became problematic, when pigs on a French military camp came down with both the Bird Flu and a human flu strain at the same time. The flu inside the pig mutated and created a super flu. This Bird Flu, after mutating, was acquired by humans and also now had the ability to transfer from human to human; the presence of a pig or bird was no longer required to obtain the flu. This resulted in the creation of the 1918 super flu. The mixing of flu's could have also happened if a human with the Bird Flu acquired another human flu concurrently, allowing the proteins to mix, resulting in the Bird Flu mutating into a human to human transferring flu. Both of these scenarios are highly possible explanations of how the 1918 flu mutated.

What can we learn from the Bird Flu of 1918, that we can apply to today's threat? As a wise man once said, *"If you are ignorant of the past you are doomed to repeat it."* We don't want to do that. Understanding the pandemic of 1918 will give us the best knowledge of what could be yet to come. What caused people to live or die? Did the people of 1918 do anything that increased or hindered their chance of survival? Studying the past flu and solving some of its riddles can translate into many lives saved today. The 1918 flu gives us clues as to what the Bird Flu's symptoms are, how rapid it can spread, who will be most affected, where it may strike first. Armed with this knowledge we can better prepare our lives.

To study the flu of 1918 we must first look for unhealthy habits in the life style of that time. Life in 1918 consisted of World War I troops being mobilized, United Service Organizations (USO's) staying open all night, smoking had become popular, and Pellagra (a vitamin B deficiency) was rampant. Each one of these factors played a role in the pandemic of 1918 becoming deadly.

## LIFE IN 1918

- **Pellagra is rampant (a vitamin B deficiency)**
- **WW I mobilization**
- **Smoking and drinking**
- **Staying up late**
- **Eating white un-enriched flour**

Pellagra was hitting the U.S. hard during the time of the 1918 flu. This is important, because Pellagra is a vitamin B deficiency. Vitamin B is a vitamin that helps the body deal with stress. The population was under a lot of stress because of WWI. A population lacking Vitamin B and under a great amount of stress would show more health related signs of stress, resulting in a greater negative impact on the immune system.

The appearance of Pellagra was probably due to the refining of flour and rice. In 1880 brown rice started to be processed into white rice. Dr. Christian Eijkman discovered experimenting with chickens, in the late 1800's, that the polishing of rice (the processing of brown rice into white rice) caused Beriberi (another name for Pellagra). His chicken experiment was proven true again by Dr. Casimir Funk in the early 1900's. By 1905 the refining process made its way to wheat. Whole wheat flour was now becoming processed white flour. This new flour had a dramatic reduction in nutrients; the loss of vitamin B being one of the casualties of the refining process. During the processing of grains, approximately 75% of the nutrients are removed, including vitamin B and many other vitamins and minerals. By 1912 white flour was commercially being produced across the country. It wasn't until the 1930's that our government ordered the replacement of the vitamin B's which were processed out of the flour. This resulted in a new product, labeled *Enriched Flour.* Unfortunately this was too late for those suffering in 1918.

In 1939 the FDA required Vitamin B to be added back into white flour: thiamine (B1), riboflavin (B2), niacin (B3). At first, companies added back into the flour the natural form of Vitamin B, shortly after which the synthetic vitamins were able to be developed inexpensively compared to the natural ones. Synthetic B soon replaced natural B vitamins in the *"enriched"* flour. The flour with the added B vitamins would bear the label *"enriched flour"*. The vitamins that were put back did not equal the amount taken out. The flour with the vitamin enrichment still had over 70% less nutrients than the original flour before processing. The 1918 American diet, containing un-enriched processed white flour, would severely lack Vitamin B. Add that to the stress the population was under, due to WWI, and you can see where the population's immune systems were headed.

A picture of what life was like then can be found in the book *Pale Horse, Pale Rider,* which is a fictional account of life in 1918; however, it is considered an excellent portrayal of life during the pandemic. *Pale Horse, Pale Rider* portrays young people in 1918 as smokers and alcohol drinkers, with a daily routine of staying up late. These activities alone would lead one to conclude that their immune systems were stressed. All of these factors (smoking, drinking and sleep deprivation) stress the immune system. Smoking alone can lead to the lungs having an inflamed condition, which could have allowed the virus to be more aggressive. Lack of sleep also lowers immunity, which may have been a factor in the health of those who died. The many men trying to get in one last hurrah by staying up late at USO's before they shipped off to war, put their bodies under stress causing sleep deprived stress. Several other minor factors could have added to the young people's suffering. These other factors could be combined, resulting in a high death rate. Pasteurization of milk could have been one of the factors, because pasteurization kills the bad and the good bacteria. A person drinking pasteurized milk could reduce the good intestinal bacteria in the body. The good bacteria promote immunity (good bacteria found in the colon produces vitamin K, a necessary blood clotting factor needed to survive the Bird Flu). The processing of rice and wheat from whole grains into white end products, removing the vital calcium (pH alkalizer) and B vitamins (known today for their calming affects) from the grains leaves the body more susceptible to stress. Vitamin B is necessary for the absorption of iron. Iron is required to oxygenate the body. Viruses do not do well in an oxygen enriched environment.

Any number of combinations of stresses could have resulted in the deaths of many. A single stress may not have killed anyone, but it is easy to see how a combination of stresses could. It would be hard to pinpoint only one stress that was the main culprit, and say *"this is the xyz stress that caused many young people's immune systems to fail."* We can only speculate that without the stresses one would have a better chance of survival.

In 1918 people lived in crowded living conditions that caused them to be more susceptible to disease. The poor had a higher death rate than the wealthy, because nurses and doctors were in short supply. Many poor did not have access to medical treatment so they died. If a person drank alcohol and was under a tremendous amount of stress they died. Was getting the virus a death sentence? Is getting the virus the only one factor that caused the disease or were there others? A combination of factors led to the deaths of thousands. Each factor alone did not guarantee a death would occur but when the factors were combined with a stimulus of stress, death occurred in record numbers. In 1918, if one or more stress factors were present, a person's chance of survival went down. It has been shown that (virus + stresses = flu).

Recall the French military base where it was believed the 1918 Bird Flu originated. What was life like there? A lot of allied troops from different nations were based together during World War I, making it easy for a disease from one nation to spread to another. Needless to say, the troops at the base were under a lot of stress. This is an important observation, since stress is one of the key factors in developing the flu. What was going on inside their bodies? How was stress affecting them? Stress causes the body's systems to increase in acidity. An acidic body condition, when fighting Bird Flu can have deadly consequences. Viruses and bacteria thrive in an acidic environment.

The troops in the U.S. before they were deployed over seas most likely had acidic bodies, because of the stress they were experiencing. If they were not heading off to war, they were training day and night, preparing for mobilization or spending way too much time at the USO's. The increased stress factors allows for illnesses to develop more easily.

When we are under stress our heart rate goes up. This is important to note, because our circulation increases. If we are bleeding, then an increased circulation would increase the amount we bleed. The quicker blood circulates, the more fluid there is to fill our lungs. Many of the people who died in 1918 died, because of fluid filling their lungs.

## FLUID FILLED THE LUNGS, BECAUSE:

- **It is an immune response to the body trying to fight off the virus**
- **Mucus is not being expelled from the lungs**
- **Blood vessels in the lungs burst causing the lungs to fill with blood**

*(The patient eventually dies of suffocation, or a complication of the flu, like pneumonia.)*

We have all heard of or experienced being a parent with a sick child. The parent is up all night caring for the child. A day or two later the parent is suffering from the same illness the child brought home. What caused the parent to get sick? Three factors were at play in this case.

## THE PARENT WAS:

- **Exposed to the virus (may have even slept in the child's room)**
- **Under mental stress from watching a child go through an illness**
- **Lacked the proper sleep required for the immune system to fight the exposure to the virus**

It was the combination **(virus + stresses = illness)** that led to the parent developing the illness, not just the mere experience of being exposed to the illness. Just as in 1918 it was a combination of stresses that led to the high mortality rate among 20-40 year old soldiers.

## IN 1918, 20-40 YEAR OLD DEATHS WERE CAUSED BY:

- **Close living quarters (virus exposure)**
- **Over exercising (physical stress)**
- **Lack of sleep (sleep deprived stress)**
- **Stress from going to war (mental stress)**
- **Pellagra (chemical stress)**
- **Smoking (chemical stress)**
- **Drinking (chemical stress)**

If a soldier just over exercised, lived in close quarters and had the stress of deployment many survived, but add smoking, drinking, staying up all night, and Pellagra; they didn't have a chance.

A young man while serving in Europe during WWI wrote home to his family:

*"If I had been a whiskey drinker, I would have been a goner."*
Private Thomas L. Roberts

Private Thomas was observant enough to notice that those who died also drank alcohol. Another example of an over stressed immune system is a man named Olf, who was in the 20-40 year old age group, whom I mentioned earlier from Crosby's book. He was strong but not healthy by any means. How do we know this? Even though he was described as a prime specimen of health, he was not healthy, but I'll let you be the judge. Olf could pick up a 180 pound man with one arm, down 25 martinis and then swim across a lake. From this description what do we know about Olf? Olf exercised a lot and was strong, but drank. Anyone who drinks 25 martinis in one sitting does not have his health under control. How did he eat? Did he smoke? Was he staying up all night partying, just before he was deployed? What we do know is he died of the flu while being transported across the Atlantic. Olf most likely was strong, but not healthy. A mistake Health Officials made in 1918 was confusing strength with health.

The unusually high death rates in the 20-40 year old age group was thought to be a mystery, because this age group usually is least affected when illnesses appear. With any illness often the very young and the very old have the highest deaths. During 1918 the rules changed. Most of the troops present on military bases were in the age group of 20-40 year olds. This is the age group of the men that were fighting the war. Since, the largest loss of life from Bird Flu in 1918 was in this age group, some health officials drew the conclusion, that since this age group has the best immune system and the most casualties, having a good immune system makes you more susceptible to dying from the Bird Flu. A theory was *"that an over immune response caused the lungs to become over inflamed and resulted in death."*

I'm not here to say that isn't true, but consider the facts. This age group was under a combination of stresses and had more unhealthy habits than any other age group; that is why they died.

The troops were also in cramped living conditions, giving them high exposure to the virus. During troop mobilizations, the buses were packed three soldiers to a seat and the trains were just as confined. The sea transports were also loaded to the gills. The filling of transports to capacity, combined with an infectious illness was a disaster waiting to happen. The illness could spread easier than soft butter.

The men returning home from the war may have been carriers for the disease. After the war was over the men went home to their wives whom, for the most part, were in the same age group. Most pregnant women are also in this age group. Pregnant women, who caught the flu in 1918, had nearly a fifty percent mortality rate. This too would cause a raise in the statistics for the 20-40 year olds.

As you can see, a logical reason exists why so many 20 to 40 year olds died. The war changed everything, causing excessive stress for the young people and, therefore, their death. Who will be our 20 to 40 year olds today? Who will the Bird Flu affect the most? What can we do to protect them and ourselves?

Your grandparents probably survived the flu of 1918 because they had healthier habits than those that didn't. They were not doing the same thing the 20-40 year olds who died were doing. Remember, Private Thomas L. Roberts wrote home from the war to say, *"If I had been a whiskey drinker, I would have been a goner."* He probably did not die because he was not drinking like some of the others his age. If you do not have bad habits today, you also will have a good chance of surviving a pandemic, just like your grand or great grandparents did.

*“The more we study,*
*the more we discover our ignorance.”*

Percy Bysshe Shelley

# 9

# 10 People The Bird Flu Will Strike The Hardest

## *A compromised immune system can put you more at risk of developing the flu*

The first thing you are going to want to do is read about who will be affected most and if it does not apply to you, you may plan to skip this section. Please don't stop reading! If you take the time to read this entire section you may discover one thing that might save your life. Even though you don't think it, at first, applies to you, you may find the information beneficial to someone you know and love. Please keep reading!

When we think of who will die or survive a disaster no one can say for sure which one we will be; however, like with all disasters, some things will make you more susceptible to illness than others. In the case of the Bird Flu there will be those most affected and those least affected. The trick here is to learn what we can do to increase our chance of survival. Science has tried to break illnesses down into simple terms, trying to find that one thing that causes death. Life does not work that way, a combination of problems lead up to a death, not one single factor. For example, if a man is shot by a bullet and dies, what caused his death? It was not the bullet that killed the man but the hemorrhaging on the operating table, or was it? Now was it the hemorrhaging or the bullet that caused the death? The fact of the matter is that the guy would not have been on the operating table, if he had not been hit by a bullet.

Can we guarantee that we won't get hit? We could even go further and say if the guy had not needed to travel an hour to the hospital he might have been saved. As you can see when we are talking about death and dying it is a combination of things that could lead to the dying. The hour ride to the hospital is not the soul factor in the death, but being hit by the bullet, the hour ride and the hemorrhaging together led to the death. We need to look at any illness as a combination of factors that resulted in the illness. The more we can reduce the amount of factors that lead up to a death, the better chance we will have that our immune system will be able to handle the problem.

If your immune system is challenged in anyway, you need to start working to build it up right now. As with any flu the very young and the very old will be greatly affected, if a Bird Flu were to arrive at anytime. The elderly that were alive in 1918, over the age of two (Children under the age of two have immune systems that are not fully developed and may not develop immunity when exposed to illnesses.), and also living in an area that was affected by the Bird Flu, may not need to worry. If the elderly were exposed to the 1918 virus and many other influenza viruses, it is possible that their immune system may have developed an immunity to the disease. The immune challenged, the senior citizens over 60, and the very young, children under the age of five, should follow the steps in the *How to Survive* section to give them the best chance of survival.

In addition to the very young, senior citizens and the immune challenged, the following information lists ten people that could be greatly affected by the Bird Flu. These types of people are not necessarily those that will, in fact, die. No one could ever say that for sure. They are those that already have one strike against them and if they keep adding strikes against their immune system they may end up dead. High risk people need to start right now preparing for the influenza. You have no time to waste. Taking steps in the right direction now could control the problem and increase your chance of survival.

# 1. OVERWEIGHT

## PROBLEM:

People that are overweight generally have reduced lung capacity, weak lungs, an acidic body condition and constipation.

Having a reduced lung capacity will allow fluid to fill the lungs more easily or have the lungs give out sooner than they should. Remember that most of those who died of the Bird Flu in 1918 died, because their lungs filled with fluid or their lungs gave out. If you are overweight and lose your breath when walking a short distance, this should be your clue that you need to work on strengthening your lungs. However, if you are not overweight but still have shortness of breath, you too will want to consider enhancing your lung's ability to overcome shortness of breath. Anyone who gets shortness of breath should work on increasing their lung capacity. The more room in your lungs to gather fluid, the more time your body has to fight the invaders. Time will be crucial when your body is fighting the virus. Your body is trying to win the war, before the lungs fill with fluid to the point of suffocation. Also, the stronger your lungs the easier it will be for them to expel fluids through coughing.

Eating a lot of refined carbohydrates will lead to a body with an overall blood acidity. Don't forget viruses tend to thrive in an acidic condition. Sugar leads to an acidic condition. Both sugar and alcohol abusers need to watch their body's pH. They both can suffer from similar illnesses, since alcohol is often cured in sugar. They both can also develop cirrhosis of the liver, which may have resulted from an acidic condition damaging the liver.

Constipation is a problem often experienced by overweight individuals. The bowels in Chinese medicine are the openings to the lungs. Keeping the bowels clear would be beneficial.

## SOLUTION:

To increase lung capacity, start with deep breathing exercises, and then work up to exercising. Remember it is important to do this under a doctor's care so that you don't over do it. (Refer to the mailbox running section for tips on how to increase lung capacity.)

A reduction in refined carbohydrate consumption would be an asset to an overweight person. Adding a lot of greens to your diet could create a more alkaline environment, which is unfriendly for viruses. If you don't like eating greens, try drinking them. Liquid Chlorophyll found in most health food stores can be mixed with water and taken as a drink. The mint flavored liquid Chlorophyll makes it even easier to get down greens, and is an enjoyable drink. There are a number of different green drinks you can try. Check with your local health food store and work on finding one you like, or you can juice the greens yourself, adding a banana and some apple juice to make it more palatable. Drinking eight 8 oz. glasses of water would also help flush toxins out of the body and aid in elimination. Some bottled waters have a higher alkalinity than others, so find the most alkaline.

Preventing constipation, by keeping the bowels clear, would be beneficial; so, fiber it up! Whenever you have an unhealthy condition in the body, it is always best to talk to your doctor. Tell him your concerns and what you are trying to accomplish (increasing lung strength, increasing elimination, eating more alkalizing foods) and I'm sure they will be happy to assist you. That is what they are there for; to aid you in staying healthy, not just to get you better once you are sick. Talk to them now before the Bird Flu hits. Talk to them now while they have the time. Make your plan of action now rather than later. Remember, there are multiple reasons that lead up to death and there are a multiple of things needed to prevent death.

## 2. LUNG CHALLENGED

### PROBLEM:

Asthmatics are people who already have trouble catching their breath. Smokers, like the asthmatic, are people whose lungs are already challenged. Since we know that smoking affects the lungs and causes cancer, a smoker's lungs may not be able to handle both the smoking and the virus. Most likely, a smoker's lungs will have difficulty surviving a virus that attacks the lungs.

A study done at the University of Oregon showed that smoking causes a loss in Vitamin E, a very important anti-oxidant. The study also found that if Vitamin C is inadequate this causes faster depletion of vitamin E. Vitamin C and B in many studies have shown to be reduced in a smoker's body. Smoking will set your body up for viruses to take hold.

### SOLUTION:

Healthy lungs will be a major factor in your surviving Bird Flu. Exercising will help most asthmatics and smokers. You should be exercising instead of smoking, if surviving is your goal. Quit now before it is too late!

Exercising and deep breathing are known for increasing lung capacity. Pottenger, a scientist known for his cat study, found that only the nutritionally deprived cats had asthma; therefore, it may be possible to increase health in asthmatics and smokers by adding mega-nutrient dense food. Air purification systems have helped many asthmatics too. If you have asthma you will want to take your doctor's advice very seriously. Doing everything your doctor tells you that could help is a must now that Bird Flu could be a threat to your health.

## 3. SLEEP DEPRIVED

### PROBLEM:

Not being able to get to sleep or to stay asleep, not allowing your body enough sleep or staying up late are all things that can lead to sleep deprived stress. A new baby in the home will result in the parents having sleep deprived stress.

Staying up partying during the flu season should be avoided. This means avoiding that New Years Eve party. Just being in a crowd will increase your chance of repeated exposure to illnesses.

## SOLUTION:

If you are in the stage of your life where you are having trouble sleeping at night, take your lack of sleep very seriously; go to a doctor. A naturopathic doctor or medical doctor can suggest things like 5-HTP, melatonin, GABA, or stress reducing meditations. Exercising can also help you sleep. You don't have to take drugs, if you don't want to; just ask for help. If you don't ask, how is your doctor going to know you want to try and solve your problem without drugs. More and more doctors are aware of alternative treatments; however, they sometimes don't tell their patients because they don't know if the patient would be open to trying natural remedies first. This is true especially if a patient comes into an office requesting a drug they read or heard about in the media. Cultivate the habit of asking for natural options first.

So you still want to go to that New Years Eve party? Take a good nap the day of the party and use the essential oil of peppermint as a breath freshener, not the candy one; it has sugar, but the essential oil. Peppermint is said to have anti-viral properties, breathing air from a crowded room as well as having peppermint on your breath may lessen your exposure; however the best idea is to skip the party altogether.

If you are a new Mom and have a brand new baby, this is the time to swallow your pride and ask for help. You will need your rest and the only way you are going to get it is with help. So, ask for help regardless of whether you think you need it or not.

## 4. ALCOHOL ABUSERS

### PROBLEM:

Remember Olf, the 25 martini drinker from 1918 and Private Thomas L. Roberts who wrote home from the war to say, *"If I had been a whiskey drinker, I would have been a goner."* This applies to you, too. Don't be a drinker. Alcohol is very acidic and depletes the body of vitamin C and B. Yes, now you have to avoid not only the New Years Eve party but the alcohol at the party too. What makes alcohol so bad is that it is cured with sugar, and since sugar is acidic, by drinking the alcohol you are making it easier for viruses to take hold.

### SOLUTION:

Avoiding alcohol could save your life. Once the threat of Bird Flu is over you can invite all your bad habits back into your life if that is what you desire. By eliminating them during a pandemic you will have a better chance of being here to enjoy a drink in the future. Be a friend to yourself; limit alcohol during the flu season; especially, if someone in your household is sick.

If you must drink you could try to balance out your system by eating alkalizing foods and drinking wheat grass. (A list of alkalizing foods can be found in the section on *The Bird Flu: 10 Simple Things You Can Do Now*). Depending on how much you drink this might help.

In Thomas Appell's book *Never Get Another Cold,* he gives two examples of clients going on a weekend partying spree and then ending up sick even though they ate alkalizing foods the rest of the time. They probably recovered better and quicker since they normally ate well, but this goes to show you that one weekend of partying can set you up for disaster. Mr. Appell has great diet advice on how not to get colds and flu's. His book is simple to understand and easy to read. It has great pictures too. A real must read for surviving the Bird Flu.

## 5. HIGHLY STRESSED / FEARFUL

### PROBLEM:

The worst thing you can do right now is read everything you can on the Bird Flu and end up scaring yourself half to death. The stress can kill you and if it doesn't the Bird Flu will take care of the rest. The fight or flight mechanism does not stop working after you leave that scary movie. It takes the body time to recover; sometimes days and weeks depending on the intensity of the fright. Being afraid won't assure you that you are going to die but if you add that to other factors it just might.

What can you do about the fear; especially, if people are dying all around you? You may end up having sleep deprived stress caused by your anxiety or fear of getting the flu.

### SOLUTION:

Assume that you may have difficulty sleeping and prepare for it. Even if you normally don't have trouble sleeping, keep the following on hand: chamomile tea, Bach Rescue remedy, Ignatia (a homeopathic remedy). These will help your body deal with stress. The important thing here is to recognize how easily you frighten and start reading now what you can do to help yourself relax. Meditation, yoga, Tai Chi and exercising are good ways to relax the body. Being able to relax in a time of stress will be the most important thing you can do. Begin now trying to find what works for you. Most victims of the Bird Flu will die within a week. Waiting is not an option.

## 6. DIABETIC

### PROBLEM:

Doctors often suggest that Diabetics receive a yearly flu shot because they are more likely to get the flu. Often Diabetics have acidic blood conditions, because of the excess sugar in their blood stream due to their constant struggle to manage their blood sugar levels with insulin. Remember an acidic body condition allows for viruses to thrive.

### SOLUTION:

The only thing that will help a diabetic is diet and exercise. Diet will be a key factor in whether a diabetic will survive. Dr. Richard K. Bernstein's book, *The Diabetes Solution,* stresses diet for both diabetic types: Type I or Type II. Diet will allow the Type I diabetic to use less insulin and the Type II diabetic, depending on how severe the Type II diabetes, may be able to completely control their diabetes with his diet.

Controlling the sugar means controlling the acid condition. Dr. Bernstein's book can be purchased at www.diabetes911.net. A diabetic since the age of 12, Dr. Bernstein gives advice on how he keeps his own Type I diabetes under control. His book has earned the reputation of being the *"Diabetic Bible."* In Dr. Bernstein's book, he gives great advice on diet and using it to control diabetes. Following Dr. Bernstein's advice will also help a diabetic control the alkalinity of the blood at the same time they are controlling their sugar. Part of his diet is to inform the diabetic about artificial sweeteners. Those cute little yellow, blue and pink packets found on the table at most restaurants. I learned from his book that the powdered form of artificial sweeteners contains both the artificial sweetener and glucose (sugar). These sweeteners should be avoided by diabetics. I never knew that.

Therefore, if you don't have diabetes and are planning to use a powdered sweetener it would be beneficial to know that the powdered artificial sweetener is considered a reduced calorie sweetener, not a sugar free one. The powdered form has 96% glucose and only 4% artificial sweetener. Since artificial sweeteners and glucose are both acid forming, it wouldn't have mattered if it contained all artificial sweetener. The only sweetener that is both not acidic and sugar free is Stevia. Stevia in the powdered form is sugar free. Even though Stevia is not approved by the FDA as an artificial sweetener. You should not let that stop you; it works well as a sweetener. Stevia is an herb and considered a supplement, not a sweetener. To limit your acid forming sweeteners you might want to at least try Stevia.

Growing a Stevia plant now insures that your family will have sweeteners during a pandemic, but remember it is ten times sweeter than sugar. Even if you don't have diabetes or have trouble with blood sugar, you could still benefit from Dr. Bernstein's advice. Most of what he suggests for the diabetic diet would be great advice for the general public to follow during a pandemic. We all could use a diet that will help us keep from having high blood sugar, a condition ripe for the virus to thrive. Following his diet will give all of us the best chance of controlling our blood sugar, thus creating a virus unfriendly body to survive the Bird Flu.

## 7. PREGNANT

## PROBLEM:

Pregnant women have a body that is under stress, a body that is trying to provide for both the mother and the developing baby. The more blood a pregnant woman has that could be deposited into her lungs, makes her more vulnerable to Bird Flu. Increased growth of the baby as the mother nears her delivery date makes it harder for the lungs to fill with air. The greatest reason for the loss of life of a pregnant woman to Bird Flu is the baby diminishing the lung's capacity. Less room in the lungs could make it fill with fluids faster, plus more blood circulating in the body, may have been a disastrous combination for pregnant women during the 1918 Bird Flu pandemic.

Remember, pregnant women had a 50% mortality rate in 1918.

## SOLUTION:

Try not to get pregnant if a pandemic is looming. If you are not willing to wait, try to plan your pregnancy so that the last two months are during June and July. June and July had the least amount of deaths and the least amount of cases of the Bird Flu. At the last part of your pregnancy you have the least lung capacity; therefore, trying to time it to when the least death rates occur will give you the best chance of surviving. Also, more doctors would be available for emergencies, if the hospitals are not filled with Bird Flu cases. Above all, eat right and make sure you take your prenatal vitamins.

# 8. WEIGHT LIFTERS AND ATHLETES

## PROBLEM:

Body builders tend to eat a lot of protein and carbohydrates as the main part of their diet to build muscle. Since protein and sugar cause an acidic condition in the body, these people may not be balancing out their pH. They should check their body's pH to make sure it is indeed alkaline and if it is not, they should try to alkalize it. Remember, though Olf in 1918 was considered in prime physical shape, he died on the transport over to WWI. Thomas Appell, the author of *Never Get Another Cold*, is also a body builder. He stresses in his book, how becoming muscular at the cost of being acidic is not worth the exchange. You may look great but be sick all the time. Anyone interested in staying healthy ought to read his book.

Athletes that are focusing on winning will also tend to over exercise so they will have the endurance to win. Is winning their competition worth developing a stressed body? While exercising is great, too much is not good for you. Over exercising, like over doing anything else, will cause a body to become stressed and acidic. The athlete, like the weight lifter, tends to eat a lot of carbohydrates in order to increase energy output. This too will cause a lower immune condition.

*"Intense exercise can cause immune deficiency."*
A. Boyum, P. Wiik
Scandinavian Journal of Immunology, Feb 1996.

**SOLUTION:**

Athletes in general need to be careful to not over do it; moderation is the key, like everything else: moderation, moderation, do everything in moderation. One way for an athlete to tell if they are over doing it is by using a basic home pH test. Many pharmacies carry pH test strips for urine. Another way for an athlete to tell if their body's pH may need adjusting is the following:

## Male Athlete

A reduction in sexual desire should be a clue that you need to investigate further and check your pH.

## Young Female Athlete

If your period has stopped or become regularly more than 33 days apart, this should be a clue to investigate further and check your pH.

*All athletes would benefit from monitoring their pH before the Bird Flu arrives. This alone could increase your chance of survival.*

## 9. DENTALLY CHALLENGED

## PROBLEM:

It is being shown more and more that dental health is playing an important role in our over all health. *Weston Price* wrote 25 scientific papers and three major books on the topic. Cavitations are a dental condition where pockets in the mouth develop as a result of a tooth extraction or a root canal. The bacteria thrive in these pockets, which causes the bone to break down. The bacteria itself is not the only problem but the toxic byproduct of the bacteria causes an acidic condition in the body, making it ripe for a virus to take hold. The toxins produced by the bacteria is said to be a thousand times more deadly than snake venom.

If you have no jaw pain and feel therefore this does not concern you, think again. I learned first hand how cavitations related to developing cancer. My cavitations were located in the site of where two of my wisdom teeth had been extracted. One hole was about as big as a quarter ( 25 cent piece ) and three quarters thick. The most important thing to note is I HAD NO PAIN, NONE AT ALL! The cavitations had not reached the nerve yet. I was left unaware of the whole problem until a Naturopathic doctor found a disruption in the meridian of my head. On further investigation with a holistic dentist, the cavitations were confirmed. If you have had a root canal or a wisdom tooth extracted and are doing everything right to get your body alkaline and nothing seems to be working, try to find out if you have a cavitation.

### SOLUTION:

Not all dentists look for cavitations, so be sure to find one that does. If your dentist does not even know what a cavitation is, chances are they won't be able to tell if you have one. One way to tell if your dentist is familiar with cavitations is to ask. *"Do you own a Cavitat machine?"* Chances are if they do, they must know what a cavitation is. Cavitations are not part of a dentist's formal training, it is knowledge they must seek out on their own. A Cavitat Machine is like a sonogram, but designed for the mouth. It is used to detect cavitations. You also may want to check on the web under *Holistic* or *Complementary Dentistry*. (See Resource section)

If you still are not sure if this applies to you and want to read further about cavitations: Morton Walker's Book, *Elements of Danger* will catch you up to speed.

## 10. HIGH CHOLESTEROL OR HEART DISEASE

### PROBLEM:

Sugar in your blood stream turns into fatty acids and then clogs your arteries, or the sugar in your blood stream is so acidic that it pulls the calcium out of your bones or veins and makes them weak. According to *Sandra Goodman*, Ph.D., in her book, *Vitamin C, the Master Nutrient,* she quotes Professor John Yudkin's study which showed that men eating high quantities of sugar were significantly at greater risk of developing heart disease than those with low sugar intakes. If this is true, than those with heart disease eat a lot of sugar, not fat, which would mean more sugar is in their blood stream. Sugar will make your body acidic and create an environment for viruses to take hold. More about acidity and pH will be discussed in the section "*How to Survive the Bird Flu.*" Book after book that I have read relating nutrition to heart disease claim that sugar, not the fat in ones diet, causes heart disease; however, this is not a fact that is well accepted by Cardiologists today.

### SOLUTION:

Some of my friends have tried the low sugar diet and found that it did dramatically lower their cholesterol more than when they were on the low fat diet.

Therefore restricting your sugar intake, if you have heart disease, will not only help prevent a heart attack but also help keep your body's environment from becoming acidic, in which the Bird Flu can thrive. Get rid of the sugar, save your heart and protect yourself from the Bird Flu. You can prove this to yourself very easily by putting yourself on a low sugar diet, not changing anything else, and watch your cholesterol numbers go down. It is not a difficult thing to prove but the results are amazing.

*"We don't see things*
*as they are*
*we see things*
*as we are."*

Anis Nin

# 10

# The Bird Flu: 10 Simple Things You Can Do Now!

If a pandemic hits, we first think that those who will survive are, of course, the healthy people. What is healthy? Who is healthy? Is it the weightlifter at the gym, the guy who meditates everyday, or the guy next door that eats vegetarian? The answer is all of them and none of them. Many things make up health, not just one. How we live our total lives will determine our health. We can eat healthy but live an over stressed life style, which leaves our body in an unhealthy state; making way for viruses to take hold.

Understanding that the threat of Bird Flu exists is just not enough. We must take an active role in insuring our survival. A healthy life style is the only thing we can count on to prevent us from dying in the event of a Bird Flu epidemic. In Crosby's book, he cites the Health Commissioner S. Copeland of New York in 1918, saying, *"Spanish Flu seldom attacks the well nourished"* and remember, Private Thomas L. Roberts wrote home the same year from the war to say, *"If I had been a whiskey drinker, I would have been a goner."* Both of these statements should inform us that even in 1918 those who ate right had the best chance of survival. Eating right is more important now than ever.

So, what does it mean to eat right? A lot of debate exists over what it means to eat right. Some may even take the Commissioners statement and think that someone obese is well nourished or if someone is physically fit they are healthy. To be well nourished and have a healthy body is about the quality of food we eat, not the quantity. Eating a lot of foods lacking in nutrients is what causes obesity. Having a strong body is not necessarily having a healthy body. Don't let the outside fool you. Eating nutrient dense foods and moderately exercising is what is called *"well nourished and healthy."* What can you do to make sure you are on the right track? First of all, make sure you do not fall into the category of those that the Bird Flu will strike the hardest. However, if you do, make the necessary changes in order to help ensure your survival. Next, start by changing a few things in your body and home that may help you survive.

Following the advice in this chapter is a great place to start. Remember, before starting any new diet or exercise program, check with your doctor to make sure it will not interfere with your medication or overall health.

## 1. STOP VIRUS AND BACTERIA: CREATE THE RIGHT BODY ENVIRONMENT

Two theories exist to explain how and why viruses are transmitted from one person to another. The theories also attempt to explain why some people's symptoms are worse than others. These theories are the *Exposure Theory* and the *Environment Theory*. (For further information regarding these theories, and how the scientist developed them, please refer to Appendix A.)

Dr. Robert Koch's *Germ Theory* or *The Exposure Theory* explains, *an illness is transmitted from one individual to another by an affected person coughing, touching or breathing on the other person.* The healthy person's exposure to the illness causes them to develop the illness. The severity of the illness depends on the amount of exposure. This theory says to prevent the illness you must prevent the exposure to that illness. Relating this idea to the Bird Flu, that means to prevent getting ill you must prevent exposure by wearing an N95 or N100 mask, wipe down possibly infected surfaces, stay out of large crowds and away from those who are ill.

The Environment Theory states, *if your body has the right conditions in the body for a virus to grow and multiply, along with being exposed to an illness, you will develop an illness.* The Environment Theory feels a combination of factors causes illness, which is what Dr. Max Von Pettenkofer stated with his theory. Depending on how environment friendly the body, the more severe the case of the illness and possibly death could occur. The Environment Theory believes that to prevent an illness a person should limit exposure, and have a non-virus friendly body environment. This will prevent a virus from multiplying in a body; therefore, prevent it from developing into a life or death illness.

So, what kind of a body environment can prevent a virus from taking hold? A body that is well nourished and has proper exercise, or a body that is alkaline and not acidic. (For more on alkalizing food, see chart in the next section) An acidic polluted condition in the body is ripe for a virus to take hold. An alkaline (clean body) condition will not allow a virus to populate easily. The fewer viruses the body has to fight, the easier it is for the immune system to overcome it and heal the body. An acidic condition in the body is caused by stress, eating acid forming foods and a clogged colon.

## A VIRUS UNFRIENDLY BODY IS:

- **not stressed**
- **fed alkalizing food**
- **exercised**
- **hydrated**
- **well rested**
- **regularly receives a lot of fiber to keep the colon clean**

Survival of the Bird Flu may come down to how well your body is prepared to meet the virus. Is your body alkaline or are you acidic?

Viruses and bacteria thrive in an acidic environment and eating foods that will encourage their growth is not wise, but eating foods that hinder a virus growth is. So you say, *"When Bird Flu comes, then I will stop eating poorly."* Remember Thomas Appell's example of a person who went out and partied on the weekend-- that normally ate well—that person went out, drank alcohol and as a result became sick. The body does not just change overnight. It takes time for the body to expel toxins, mucus and change chemistry, so you need to start making changes right now. Plenty of books on changing your pH and diet exist. Find one that works for you now, rather than later. You don't want to be reading a book trying to figure out what works for you and trying to collect the things needed for survival during a pandemic. By then it is too late! Start Now!!!!

## 2. MAINTAIN AN ACCEPTABLE BODY pH

Since viruses and cancers thrive in an acidic condition and elevated glucose levels suppresses the immune system, maintaining an alkaline environment is key to surviving a Bird Flu.

To maintain an alkaline pH you must avoid acid forming foods and drinks such as soft drinks, alcohol, coffee, sugar, meat, dairy, fats and processed foods. A small portion of the population (about 8%) will have an over alkaline body state which is no better than an over acidic state. The body should maintain an alkaline balance of 6.0 - 7.5, (depending on the body fluid being tested: blood 7.35-7.45, saliva 6.0-7.5, urine 4.5-8.4), in order to stay free of a virus friendly situation. Notice that urine can have a much lower pH than any of the other body fluids. We should strive to be on the alkaline side of the spectrum (alkaline is the higher number of the range), if we are trying to prevent illness. The more alkalized the body is, the better chance it has of not experiencing an illness altogether, unless it is over alkalized. Being on the more acidic side of the acceptable alkaline range may cause us to get the disease but not to die from it. An acidic body, not at all in the acceptable range, means we are prone to illness. The more prone we are to illness, the more we need to be concerned with being exposed to the illness. The less prone your body is to a virus means fewer viruses to multiply and death is less likely to occur. Your immune system will have a better chance of combating and winning against fewer viruses.

Avoid foods that are acid forming, like sugar, meat, dairy, fats and processed foods. Foods that are alkalizing are simply the good old fruits, vegetables and whole grains. Some foods are more alkalizing than others. During a pandemic you might want to stock up on alkalizing foods:

## ALKALIZING FOODS

- Almonds
- Asparagus
- Avocados
- Beets
- Broccoli
- Brussels Sprouts
- Cabbage
- Carrots
- Celery
- Chard
- Cucumbers
- Eggplant
- Garlic
- Legumes
- Lemons
- Lettuce
- Limes
- Liquid Chlorophyll
- Olive oil
- Onions
- Peas
- Peppers
- Pumpkins
- Squash
- Spinach
- Tomatoes
- Turnips

Cooking changes the pH of a lot of foods, like tomatoes; therefore, to maintain the alkalinity of the food it is best if they are eaten raw. Raw nuts should be soaked overnight before eating for the most health benefit.

You should not limit your diet to just alkalizing foods but foods that help the body burn sugar, such as foods high in Biotin. Biotin helps in the burning of glucose by producing glucokinase, a liver enzyme, needed for sugar and fat processing. A key that biotin is great for maintaining blood sugar is that it also is known to improve glucose tolerance in some diabetics. We should not only be eating alkalizing foods but foods high in biotin.

## FOODS HIGH IN BIOTIN

- **Brewer's Yeast or Nutritional Yeast**
- **Brown Rice**
- **Liver**
- **Oats**
- **Peanut Butter**
- **Soy**

If you decide to get peanut butter, look for one without sugar or hydrogenated oils. Brown rice is a key ingredient in our electrolyte formula because of its biotin content. (For further information see *"Simple Things You Can Do Now" number eight - Folk Remedy for Balancing Electrolytes).*

## 3. TAKE VITAMINS AND SUPPLEMENTS

## VITAMINS

We have already discussed that taking vitamins if you smoke is a good idea, but taking vitamins is a good idea for everyone. Check with your doctor, if you are taking any medications, before embarking on any vitamin regiment. Ask your doctor if any of these will interfere with any medications you are taking, or any medical condition you might have before you start.

What type of person needs to supplement their diet? If you eat a lot of sugar or white flour, smoke tobacco, have frequently taken antibiotics and don't get regular sunshine, then this is the section for you. Even if you don't do any of the above, taking vitamins could strengthen your immune system. Helping your body stay healthy will increase your chance of surviving a pandemic.

Vitamin C and calcium are two of the many things used in our bodies for vein strength and health. Since Bird Flu can cause blood vessels in the lungs to burst, resulting in the lungs filling up with blood, having strong veins might increase your chances of survival. Be careful, Vitamin C can cause a body to become more acidic, creating a condition in which viruses can thrive. What should you do? Keep taking your Vitamin C? Yes! The solution is to take Vitamin C together with calcium. Since calcium helps a body to become more alkaline and strengthens veins, taking calcium in conjunction with vitamin C can balance a body's pH.

*Where to obtain quality vitamin and herbal supplements refer to the Resource section in the back of the book.*

## VITAMINS - A MUST TO HAVE ON HAND:

- **Vitamin C**
- **Calcium**
- **Magnesium**
- **Vitamin D**
- **Vitamin B**
- **Vitamin K**
- **Zinc**

The following information is adapted from *The Vitamin, and Health Encyclopedia, revised* by Jack Ritchason, N.D.

**VITAMIN C** - increases vein health. Remember during Bird Flu capillaries in the lungs burst causing the lungs to fill with fluid, suffocating the sick person. Taking vitamin C will increase vein health and possibly prevent capillaries from bursting. Vitamin C taken with calcium will help the body absorb the calcium and also reduce the acidity of the vitamin C.

**CALCIUM** - is your body's alkalizer. It helps change the body from an acid pH to an alkaline pH body condition, which viruses cannot survive. When someone is taking antacids they are in fact taking a product containing calcium. Antacids contain calcium not just because it is good for you but because the calcium helps neutralize the acid in the stomach. Don't plan on getting your calcium from your antacid. There is not enough calcium in the product to help with an acidic body condition. All calcium supplements are not alike. Some are easier for the body to use than others. The best form of calcium is chelated calcium, or Isotonic calcium. Chelated Calcium made with calcium as calcium lactate, phosphate, or citrate is easiest to absorb. Isotonic Calcium combined with Vitamin D, Magnesium and Boron helps with absorption. Isotonic Calcium that is made with fructose is the easiest to get children to take.

Coral Calcium is another calcium the body can easily utilize; however, some unscrupulous companies do not harvest the coral calcium properly, thus rendering it almost useless. Look for a brand harvested from the reef beds, not above water. If the coral calcium is harvested above water, the minerals and life supporting elements are often leached out by the sun. Coral calcium's do not have a high volume of calcium compared to other calcium supplements; however, their natural formulation does alkalize the body quickly.

According to my research, the calcium's' to avoid are calcium carbonate and oyster shell calcium. These are indeed calcium, but they are difficult for the body to absorb and utilize. Calcium's that are laced with sugar are also pointless; since sugar pulls calcium out of the body at the same time you are trying to put it back into the body. Sugar also makes a body acidic while you are trying to alkalinize it. Avoid calcium supplements that contain white sugar, unless they are made from fructose and intended for children. Children's calcium supplements often require sugar in some form to make it more palatable. Try to use children's supplements that use fructose rather than sucrose for sweetening. Fructose is less acidic than sucrose.

**MAGNESIUM AND VITAMIN D** - both help your body absorb calcium; they too might be something to consider adding to your vitamin regiment. Getting 15 to 20 minutes of sunlight a day should be enough vitamin D to aid in calcium absorption. Vitamin D is often obtained from the sun or found in fish oils. Magnesium can be found in whole grains, dark green vegetables, nuts, seeds and brown rice.

**VITAMIN K** - will be an important vitamin for the Bird Flu. Vitamin K is made by the beneficial bacteria in your colon and aids in blood clotting. We want our blood to be able to clot if our capillaries burst during the Bird Flu. Many women after giving birth are given a vitamin K shot to prevent hemorrhaging. Wouldn't it be great if your body could provide enough vitamin K without a shot during the Bird Flu? If you have taken antibiotics periodically, you are in great need of beneficial bacteria. Some grocery store products claim to contain beneficial bacteria, which could help you build good bacteria in your colon. You can find a beneficial bacteria (probiotics) supplement, such as acidophilus in most health food stores. Probiotics like acidophilus and bifidophilus for the greatest viability should be found in your health food store's refrigerator section and not on the shelf. Once you get it home, probiotics should be kept in the refrigerator, to maintain their continued viability until the expiration date listed on the product. If the probiotic is taken right before bedtime, it will have the best chance of taking up residence in your colon and providing you with the vitamin K you are seeking.

**VITAMIN B** – helps the body cope with stress, creating an oxygen environment (red blood cells depend on them). Where can we find them? In whole grains, most vegetables, dairy products and molasses. Whole grains are rich in vitamin B, however they can be acidic and mucus forming in nature. But, wait, don't throw them out with the bath water, this would be ridiculous. Since stress is going to be a major factor in developing the Bird Flu, and whole grains have vast amounts of vitamin B, we need them. Think of trying to balance your diet instead of avoiding any and all acid and mucus forming foods. A good balanced diet will keep our pH in balance. Using anti-mucus herbs will help prevent mucus build up. Keep in mind, since grains can be acidic and cause mucus, we do not want to eat too much, but we do want to balance them in our diet with green vegetables or alkalizing foods. Dairy can be mucus forming too and should be limited.

**ZINC** - We all know zinc is great for colds and flu's but did you know it is also great for insulin metabolism; therefore, taking zinc will help in two ways: by assisting with the flu and by reducing sugar in the blood.

Many other anti-oxidants exist. The above vitamins are not the only ones you can have on your shelf. You might want proanthocynanidins, or even natural vitamin E. The above are the bare minimum to have on hand for a pandemic.

## SUPPLEMENTS

- **Capsicum**
- **Olive Leaf**
- **Mullein**
- **Cherry Bark**
- **Horehound**
- **Slippery Elm**
- **Liquid Chlorophyll**
- **Echinacea and Goldenseal**

The following information is adapted from *The Little Herb Encyclopedia,* also by Jack Ritchason, ND. In the event the Bird Flu leaves you with no other alternatives for survival, these herbs may save your life.

Herbs and Products can be purchased at your local health food store or online at escaperthebirdflu.com

**CAPSICUM** – is the most important supplement you can have on your shelf. It has antibacterial, diaphoretic, hemostatic and antiseptic properties, which means in plain English that it fights infection, causes sweating, stops bleeding, combats viruses and bacteria, thus preventing infection.

**OLIVE LEAF, ECHINACEA AND GOLDENSEAL** are virus and infection fighters. You may not need all three. This winter, try to find which one works best for you and your family, by using it now before you really need it.

**MULLEIN, CHERRY BARK AND HOREHOUND** are mucus reducers. Since mucus and blood are the two fluids that fill the lungs, leading to suffocation, preventing one or both of them will reduce the amount of fluids in the lungs. These herbs reduce the mucus by breaking the mucus up, thereby making it easier to expel. When mucus is easier to expel, the coughing to expel it will be less intense. When the coughing is less intense less blood vessels will burst. This may help prevent excess fluids, resulting in suffocation. Simply put, less mucus in the lungs equals less fluid in your lungs. Once again, you may not need all of these herbs. Try one or two this winter to find out which one works best for you.

**SLIPPERY ELM BARK** is often found in bulk form, rather than in a pill. All dried herbs are usually prepared by making a tea.

## SLIPPERY ELM TEA

**1 tsp Slippery Elm Herb**

**1 Cup Water**

1) **Bring a pot of water to a boil**
2) **Remove it from the heat**
3) **Add Slippery Elm herb**
4) **Let seep with cover on for 20 minutes**
5) **Strain and drink**

Slippery Elm is an herb that is so soothing on a sore throat that you will definitely want to have it on hand. It can be ordered online at escapethebirdflu.com or from *Frontier* (see *Resource Section* for more information).

**LIQUID CHLOROPHYLL** is found in abundance in most green vegetables and is a must have herb. If you don't eat green vegetables take chlorophyll in a liquid or pill form. It is always best to get it from your food, but if you can't, or won't, this is a close second. Chlorophyll has a lot of iron and helps develop red blood cells in the body. Developing healthy blood will insure adequate oxygen in the body. Once again, viruses do not do well in an oxygenated environment.

## COMBINATION FORMULAS

- **Airborne**
- **Oscillococcinum**
- **Target P14**

**AIRBORNE** is a cold and flu remedy that was invented by a teacher. It has been shown to be quite effective in preventing the flu. What is nice about *Airborne* is that they have a product designed especially for children. *Airborne* can be found at your local drugstore.

**OSCILLOCOCCINUM** is a homeopathic flu combination made by Boiron. It may be found in your local drug store right next to *Airborne.*

**TARGET P14** is an herbal combination by Nature Sunshine, a supplement company that has developed a product called *"Target P-14,"* that has been used by diabetics to help control their blood sugar. My research reveals that this product could be beneficial in surviving the Bird Flu.

The following ingredients are listed on the bottle and the definitions are adapted from *The Little Herb Encyclopedia,* by Jack Ritchason, ND

## TARGET P14

**CAPSICUM** - fights infection, causes sweating, stops bleeding, combats and neutralizes viruses & bacteria, prevents infection
**CEDAR BERRIES** - stop bleeding, pain
**CHROMIUM** - sugar metabolism
**DANDELION** - toxin elimination, feeds intestinal flora, reduces inflammation and muscle spasm, pH alkalizer
**GARLIC** - fights respiratory, infections, increases immune response, expectorant
**JUNIPER BERRIES** - fights infections, reduces inflammation
**LICORICE** - reduces pain and inflammation, phlegm expelling, strengthens adrenal glands
**MARSHMALLOW** - good for bronchial asthma, shortness of breath, wheezing, respiratory complaints
**MULLEIN** - reduces inflammation, relieves chronic coughing, pain relief

**NETTLE** - stops bleeding, lowers blood sugar
**SLIPPERY ELM** - soothes irritation of mucus membranes, balances intestinal flora
**UVA URSI** - soothes tightened and inflamed tissue
**WHITE OAK BARK** - shrinks tissue & constricted blood vessels, reduces bleeding and mucus, strengthens veins
**YARROW** - shrinks inflamed tissue, stops bleeding, induces sweating, relaxes muscle spasms, pH alkalizer
**ZINC** - helps with insulin metabolism

## 4. LEARN TO COOK FROM A RECIPE

While my sister was reading a magazine in France, she came across a startling statistic: only 10% of the U.S. women cook from a recipe on a regular basis. I don't know how accurate that statement is, but I'm sure it is pretty close to being true. My sister further joked, *"And you are probably in the 1% that cooks from wheat berries."* Okay, so I make my own flour and then cook from a recipe. I love it and it works for me. Cooking from a recipe is becoming a lost art. I learned to cook from my grandmother; my own mother rarely cooked from a recipe. If our economic infrastructure were to ever fail it most likely will fail big. Our food delivery infrastructure is insufficient to handle a disaster because every company is trying to cut costs. This cost reduction has all companies streamlining with very little failsafe measures left intact. When the Katrina Hurricane hit New Orleans our shelves in Florida became bare. I had never seen such empty shelves. For instance, bananas that normally came through New Orleans Ports were scarce on the shelves here in Florida.

Storing food for a pandemic is going to be a must. Packaged foods take up much more room than if the ingredients were to be stored separate. Also, if companies fail, we may have to go back to the old way of doing things before things get back on track.

Learn to cook now! If you won't, try reading a cookbook on your own or watch a Saturday cooking show. At the very least make sure you have a good Betty Crooker Cookbook, and learn to use it.

Learning to cook from a recipe will be impossible during a pandemic, because there are so many spices and other ingredients needed for basic cooking that you may not have thought of stocking before. If you could just learn to make one meal from a recipe, let it be soups and biscuits. Many a pioneer family survived the winter on soups. Most recipes require some key ingredients. These ingredients are absolute musts every pantry should have if you plan to cook from a recipe.

## PANTRY INGREDIENTS FOR PREPARING RECIPES

- **Powdered Milk**
- **Powdered butter**
- **Powdered eggs**
- **Salt**
- **Baking soda**
- **Grains or Flour**
- **Sweetener**
- **Flavorings and spices**

The powder ingredients will last for a long time and don't require refrigeration. Salt and baking soda make things like cookies, pancakes and biscuits rise. Grains or flour will work as filler for a meal in the form of biscuits and pancakes. Sweetener makes things taste better. Keep in mind you want **value based sugars,** like molasses, stevia, brown sugar or honey. These sweeteners not only are sweet but also provide nutrition as well. Also, keep on hand, flavorings such as bullion for soups, vanilla for cookies, herbs and spices like oregano and seasoned salt. Depending on your taste and needs you will want to have many different flavorings and spices.

## 5. GET A HOME AIR PURIFIER

On a talk show the CDC suggested that you purchase a filtering mask, either the N95 or N100. The problem with obtaining a mask is that the first time you use it; it may become contaminated and should be thrown away. If the Bird Flu lasts 18 months, like it did in 1918, and you just went out once a week, you would require 78 masks for one person. If you have more than one person, the number of masks you would need would go up. Mask ownership may be a good start but is there more you can do?

What about air purifiers, can they help? Yes, they can. What should you look for? An air purifier is not an air filter; there is a difference. An air filter requires the air go through it in order for it to clean the air. The air in the far end of the room has the least chance of becoming clean since the fan usually is not powerful enough to draw the far reaching air to the machine. An air purifier changes the make up of the indoor air by adding ozone and charged ionization to restore the air quality inside to what is found naturally in outdoor air.

Our outside air, according to Al Gore in his movie *An Inconvenient Truth,* is containing less and less oxygen and more CO2. Since viruses live better in less oxygen, this could be a growing problem. We also spend time inside our home breathing out CO2, creating an environment with even less oxygen than what is found naturally outside. Our indoor air becomes stagnant and uncharged. The air outdoors has both negative and positive charged ions. Air purification's goal is to restore the inside air quality to outside standards. The one that I have found to be most effective is a brand called Natural Air (see Appendix B).

My research revealed that viruses, bacteria and cancer survive better in a less oxygenated environment and since oxygen is a byproduct of ozone, it might help to increase the oxygen in the indoor environment to prevent viruses and bacteria.

The N95 or N100 cloth masks recommended by the CDC, to help control the spread of the virus, can be placed in front of the machine for one hour and then turned over to kill many, if not all of the viruses that may have come in contact with the mask.

Will it kill all the viruses? We do not know since it has not been tested, but your only other option is to have a mask for every person every day, for 18 months. Individual masks can cost up to $40.00 each. For one person, going out once a week for a year and a half, the costs for masks would be 40 x 78 = $2,800.00 and even more if the person went out more than once a week. A machine by Natural Air retails for $399.99, for a savings of about $2,400.00 your whole family would benefit. You will still need to have on hand several masks per person, but you should not require as many masks as you would without the machine, since you will be able to reuse them. With an air purification machine you would not have to worry about running out of masks, since you have a way of recycling them. You still might want to purchase a mask for as many outings as you can, but not knowing the length of time the Bird Flu will be around, having an air purification system would give you the security that you might be able to reuse the masks if push comes to shove. Will an air purifier guarantee that you will not get the Bird Flu? Based on my research they will at least give you a fighting chance at being less exposed to the virus.

## 6. EXERCISE

Exercising is more important now than ever. Why? Exercising will reduce your stress level. This will keep your body alkaline and in turn will ward off disease. Exercising will also strengthen your lungs, which will help prevent them from failing due to exhaustion, if you do acquire the Bird Flu.

Before starting any new diet, or exercise program, check with your doctor to make sure it will not interfere with your medication or overall health. You may need to begin with deep breathing, working your way to walking, before you begin a more aggressive exercise program.

Earlier when we talked about stress we said, due to the fight or flight response, stress causes elevated cortisol and sugar in the blood. Exercising will help the body use the sugar in the blood that was released from the fight or flight stress response. Since a lot of stress is associated with people dying during a pandemic, exercising is one way of keeping that stress under control.

Cardiovascular exercise is a way of getting the lungs ready for an assault. The Bird Flu affects the lungs. When the lungs are exercised by deep breathing and cardiovascular exercise they will be better equipped to handle excessive coughing brought on by the Bird Flu. Many of the people died in 1918, because their lungs gave out from all the coughing to remove the excessive phlegm in their lungs.

Mailbox running is a technique I developed to help me exercise my lungs (see the section on Mail Box Running in 10 Steps). Before developing mailbox running, I tried a local walking trail until it was closed for repairs. I then tried to run on a fitness path, where I had run the previous year until an alligator visited the area. On my next attempt at running on the fitness path, I found a water moccasin in the middle of the path, so I waited until another day and tried again and found another (or the same snake) under a tree resting a foot and a half off the path.

Out of frustration, mailbox running was created. Not being an avid runner I wanted to start slowly and work my way up without forcing the issue. Mailboxes are the key. I began by getting in my car, taking down the mileage and driving a half mile to find my turn around point. I observed the nearest mailbox and made that mailbox my midway marker and turn around point. It was easy to remember, since almost everyone on my street has a different mailbox style. The next morning I began running. I started running on the right side of my street, running with the flow of traffic and soon learned to switch to running on the other side of the street. I changed sides, because my street led out of the housing area and so did a lot of people in their cars heading off to work. I was headed in the same direction towards the housing development's exit to the main road, which left me breathing in a lot of car fumes. Yuck! Running on the left side, I avoided breathing in the fumes from the cars as people left for work.

My first day, I set a realistic goal and tried to run as far as I could without over doing it. I did not make my goal but remembered the mailbox where I stopped running and walked until I reached my midway mailbox. Turning around, staying on the same side of the street, I began running again, setting a realistic goal and not quite meeting that goal either. Once again, remembering the mailbox where I stopped, I ended my run and walked home. My goal from that point on was to meet my previous days running mark for the rest of the week. The next week I set my goal to run one mailbox further than I did the previous week.

I developed mailbox running, because I hate running. This method helped me to see progress in my running and is rather painless. After all, it is only one more mailbox, not another mile. I run four to five days a week. By Friday I find myself saying, *"I know I can make that next mailbox."* I hold off running to it, so on Monday I will have the confidence that I can make it and will want to get up and prove it to myself.

On Monday when I make it to my target mailbox, it makes a good start for my week. At times I stop just short of reaching my goal on Tuesday or Wednesday. In Florida I run later in the evening, or early in the morning to avoid the heat. The hotter it is the harder it is for me to make my goal. If I have not slept well or eaten right the day before, it will always be harder for me to reach my goal. I don't let the days I fall short get me down, because I have found that by the end of the week I have met my goal more often than not. The point here is not to give up. Take it one day at a time.

If you are not fit enough to begin running, begin walking as far as you feel comfortable, turning around and walking home. Add a mailbox each day until you reach your half mile mailbox. Then begin running to the first mailbox and walking 'til the half way mailbox turnaround point and run to the first mailbox and walk the rest of the way home. Add a mailbox a week until you can run the whole mile.

If even walking is a problem, then begin by doing deep breathing exercises for five minutes a day, adding a minute or two each week until you think you can begin walking to your mailbox and back into the house. The next day walk to your neighbor's mailbox and back. Each week add a mailbox.

Andrew Weil has a great CD, as I mentioned before, called *Breathing, the Master Key to Self Healing.* Using his tape will help you increase your lung capacity.

The point here is to begin with something and work your way up slowly so you can stick to it. Make sure when you exercise you do not over do it to the point of exhaustion, because that will put more stress on your body than it will help. Going slowly makes it easy. The key is sticking to it and not giving up.

Cardiovascular exercise is a great exercise for your lungs and reduces blood sugar. Keeping your lungs exercised will keep them healthy and prepared to fight the Bird Flu. Just don't over do it. The Bird Flu may be a war you have no choice but to fight.

## MAILBOX RUNNING IN 10 STEPS

1. **Determine the ½ mile midway mailbox**
2. **Run or walk on the left side of the street, if heading towards the housing development entrance, or the right side, if headed to the back of your housing development.**
3. **Set a realistic goal and begin running, attempting to meet your goal**
4. **Notice the marker mailbox (mailbox where you stopped running). Make it your goal to reach the marker mailbox the next day.**
5. **Walk the rest of the way to the midway mailbox and turn around.**
6. **Repeat step 3: only this time you are running home. Set a realistic goal and begin running to meet your goal.**
7. **Notice the return home marker mailbox (mailbox where you stopped running) and finish walking home. This mailbox is now your goal for tomorrow.**

8. **Maintain running to these two marker mailboxes for the rest of the week.**

9. **Next week your goal will be the mailbox past your marker mailbox.**

10. **After reaching your goal of running two separate half-mile increments, try to run a full mile. Only one marker mailbox is needed. Continue until you can run the full mile, and then try to improve your running time.**

It may be necessary to adjust how many mailboxes you add per day, depending on how close the mailboxes are in your neighborhood. If you are living in a townhouse area you may want to add two mailboxes. If the mailboxes are grouped together, you might want to take the time to paint a spot on the road every fifty feet. Use a different color for your turn around point. If you live in a rural area, paint a spot on a tree, every fifty feet, or use fence posts, adding a certain number every week. The point here is to find a way of adding a little more to your running every week until you meet your goal. Good luck! And don't give up! Consistency is the key.

## 7. REDUCE EXPOSURE

Viruses thrive in certain conditions, just like animals, people, plants and most living things. The better our living environment and the more food we have, the more we reproduce. In the wild, if food is scarce, animals will have smaller families; just like viruses, if they have less favorable environments they will grow and multiply more slowly. Sugar creates a condition favorable for viruses to grow. In the following example I will show you why you will want to reduce your exposure to viruses. The fewer viruses your body is working to kill at one time, the more time it will have to develop antibodies to keep the viruses under control.

Reducing exposure to the illness is your first line of defense.

Think of your body as a kitchen with only a few specks of food left out. A few cockroaches may be attracted to the food. If you leave out a bunch of food, you will be breeding cockroaches in your kitchen. It's the same way with your body. Some exposure will be a challenge for your immune system, but continual bombardment on your body may overwhelm the entire system to the point of developing the flu.

To limit exposure, stay out of crowds, or wear a N95 or N100 mask; wash your hands and avoid touching your eyes, mouth or nose. These are the things you can do in the beginning. Once Bird Flu hits, it is very important to stay away from crowds. In 1918 the highest death rates during the pandemic in Philadelphia, followed a parade and rally supporting the war effort. If you do plan to go out into a crowd, wear a mask. Remember the mask will be considered contaminated. Upon returning home after the event, the mask should not be taken inside. It should be removed with great care. How are you going to do that? Use a glove, or a rag to remove the mask by sticking your fingers inside the mask, touching it as little as possible. After removing the mask, always ***wash your hands*** before touching anything in your home. This is a must!!!!!! Use one hand to remove and throw away the mask and the other to open the door, going directly to the sink to wash your hands.

Clothes should be immediately washed, with the hands being washed again after removing the clothes. Be sure to take off masks and clothing (by turning them inside out) in such a way as to not contaminate the hands when you take them off. The outside of the mask and your clothes will be contaminated!!!!!!!!

Eco Quest makes a personal air purification system called a *Buddy*. The *Buddy* is an ionizer that hangs around the neck and, because of its design, repels foreign bodies such as allergens. There are no claims that it works on viruses, but my family used two on the plane when the SARS virus scare was in full force while we were traveling abroad. When we arrived at my sister's in England her family was sick. We continued to have our *Buddies* close by while we slept. We then traveled to the south of France to visit my other sister and her family. They too had been sick. We once again continued wearing our *Buddies* and left them on in the room while we slept. No one in my family got sick the entire trip.

## 8. DRINK WATER

What we drink can make our body sick or healthy. Drinking coffee, soda, alcohol, pasteurized milk and pasteurized juice can make our bodies acidic. If a pandemic is looming or if you get the flu, avoid these things, especially while you are ill. Remember drinks like coffee act as diuretics which cause your body to lose water and milk promotes mucus formation. Eliminating acid forming foods and drinks while you are going through an illness will help your body fight off a virus. Drinking water will help your body purge the toxins that benefit the viruses, helping them to multiply and survive. Water will reduce the toxins and slow down the duplication of the virus, giving the body more time to develop antibodies to fight off the virus. Do not think more is better. Drinking too much water can flood your cells and throw off your electrolytes. Stick to the most commonly recommended eight 8 oz. glasses of water a day. If you are sick with vomiting, diarrhea, expelling of mucus and loss of fluids due to sweat, it is necessary to replenish your electrolytes.

A simple home remedy is found below. I am offering you this remedy not to sway you from using the commercial brands but to give you something you can do just in case the commercial brands of electrolyte drinks are not available during the pandemic.

This remedy is adapted from a remedy given to me by an herbalist. She said her father who was a doctor in the early 1900's used it all the time when they were kids. It is similar to other home electrolyte formulas, except that it uses brown rice as a sugar instead of white sugar. The folk remedy electrolyte formula I feel is better, because brown rice contains essential vitamins and nutrients that will support health and white sugar does not. I have changed the original folk remedies that called for sugar to Stevia, since Stevia is more alkalizing.

## FOLK REMEDY FOR BALANCING ELECTROLYTES

1 cup brown rice

1 potato with skin left on

3 cups water

1 teaspoon of baking soda

1 packet of Stevia

1. Dice potato and put in with rice and water
2. Cook rice and potato, bringing to a boil
3. Continue cooking on medium heat for 15 minutes
4. Strain liquid into a glass
5. Add 1 teaspoon of baking soda
6. Add Stevia (an herb that is 10 times sweeter than sugar and not acidic)
7. Drink

This will not taste particularly good, but neither do the commercial ones. This however, will supply the body with needed nutrients and help the body stay hydrated. The baking soda is needed for its salt and at the same time it alkalizes the body. If you need more fluid after cooking the rice, add ½ cup of water to the rice and mix well before straining.

Using a commercial electrolyte mixture or a homemade one is not the issue; the key here is to keep the ill person's body hydrated and alkaline.

A drink that will help alkalize the body, preparing it for the Bird Flu, is a mint flavored liquid chlorophyll. A teaspoon added to 8 ounces of water is quite refreshing. Drinking liquid chlorophyll alkalizes the body and aids the body in healing. Chlorophyll helps with the body's intake of oxygen, since it is loaded with iron, but unlike iron supplements, it will not cause constipation.

## 9. GET PLENTY OF SLEEP

Not getting enough sleep will stress the body and lower its immune system. The body cleans while we are asleep. We know this since upon rising we need to use the bathroom. Our body is dumping its waste. Upon rising in the morning, it is best to eat fruit, drink water and take vitamin C. The fruit and vitamin C will help the body release toxins (by making us have a bowel movement). The fruit is filled with fiber and vitamin C, the water will flush out the toxins and the extra Vitamin C will act as a laxative--if taken to bowel tolerance--to clean out the bowels (Bowel tolerance - taken until your stools are very soft, but are not watery).

Sleep allows the body to clean and rejuvenate. A well rested body is one more capable of fighting off a viral assault. It is worth repeating that a lack of sleep will result in the body suffering from sleep deprived stress. Sleep deprived stress is derived from not getting the needed rest the body requires for maintaining health. In Hans Selye's studies he noticed a connection between an increase in adrenal gland activity and a decrease in the immune system. Which basically means the more stressed you are the more your immune system is hindered. Selye's research has been confirmed by modern immunology studies.

*"... researchers in the emerging field of behavioral immunology are beginning to explain how psychological events can affect physical health."*

Steven F. Maier, Mark Laudenslager,
Psychology Today, August 1985

Sleep deprived stress is the result of staying up late, not being able to get to sleep, or awaking in the middle of the night. Lack of sleep lowers immunity which could be a factor in getting or not getting the Bird Flu.

5-HTP, GABA, melatonin are all supplements that can help you get to sleep and stay asleep. If you are severely stressed these may not even help; however, the sleep you do get will be a better quality of sleep, then you would have received otherwise.

Once again, I can't stress it enough, if you are on any medication or have any health concerns please check with your doctor first.

Avoid bad news. Watching the *"News"* every day during a crisis time will set you up to have your fight or flight mechanism turned on, affecting your cleansing sleep. Try not to watch the News every day. Use the internet to keep up with basic information. Watching stressful News during a pandemic may cause you to have sleepless nights. Limit your exposure to disturbing News and definitely shelter your children from hearing the News. Even the slightest disturbing News may frighten a young child. The News of people dying of the Bird Flu, even though it is half a world away, may be confusing to a child. They may be thinking that people are dying in their hometown and not understand that it may be in a third world country on the other side of the globe. Kids have trouble understanding the News so keep it from them, if you can.

Get seven to eight hours of sleep. If you have children, they need at least eight to ten hours of sleep. Make sure your toddlers and younger children get that, plus. Sleep will be a key to helping your immune system fight an illness.

## 10. REDUCE STRESS / MEDITATE

Prepare yourself to reduce stress before the Bird Flu by asking yourself these questions:

## ASK YOURSELF:

- **Am I having trouble sleeping?**
- **Do I feel anxious?**
- **Is my hair falling out?**
- **Do I anger easily?**
- **Do mosquitoes love me?**

Answering *"yes,"* to any of the above questions means you should consider a stress reduction protocol. Some of the stress reducers we have already mentioned, but here is a more complete list:

## STRESS REDUCERS:

- **Yoga**
- **Meditate**
- **Prayer**
- **Exercise**
- **Work less**
- **More sleep**
- **Better diet**
- **Take a News Break**
- **Laugh as much as you cry**
- **Breathing exercises**
- **Do what relaxes you**
- **Get your affairs in order**

Yoga, meditation and prayer are useful stress reducers. Yoga relaxes the body. Meditation and prayer relaxes the mind.

There are many studies that have shown the power of prayer. Praying can be a way your mind can take a break from what ails you, giving it a chance to concentrate on something else.

I used a set of prayer beads (Catholic Rosary) to help keep my mind focused on prayer when I faced the loss of my mother, while undergoing breast cancer treatment. The Rosary gave me a focal point and a sense of peace, allowing my mind to escape the fear and frustration of the day.

If you are having difficulty praying, try repeating a prayer, or sequence of prayers, over and over again. By concentrating on what each phrase in the prayer means, this can give you a moment of peace. Praying this way will give your mind something to concentrate on without fear getting in the way. In my book, *A Journey Through Cancer,* I detail the way I relied on the Rosary to pray, when I was stressed out the most. The point here is not to get caught up in the action of praying, but to give your mind a chance to rest in the midst of chaos. In essence, by praying in this way you are giving your fears to God and your mind a chance to rest. There are a number of meditation CD's available on the market, that will guide you through a meditation. Marianne Williamson has a great *Morning and Evening meditation* Audio. There are many other meditation tapes out there but Marianne's is by far my favorite.

Getting your affairs in order will give you some peace of mind when a pandemic hits; at least, you will know there is a plan for your children, in the event of your death. Many children became orphaned, because of the unexpected number of people dying from the flu, this overwhelmed the city of Philadelphia Health's Department.

The more you are prepared, the better chance that your wishes will be done. During a pandemic your wishes could get lost in the shuffle.

***My Life in a Box,*** by Laurie Ecklund Long, is a short easy to read 32 page work book that will make getting your affairs in order a whole lot easier. Her book is considered an Emergency Preparedness Resource. Ms. Long's book is not just for Emergencies. It is a must for everyone, because you never know when your family will need the information in the event of your death. Use the Bird Flu as an excuse to organize your life for the ones you love.

A body under stress will have negative health consequences unless the stress is managed. Meditation, yoga, prayer, diet, and exercising in moderation play a role in managing stress levels. We could have stressful life situations, but by reducing stress with yoga, meditation and prayer, we can still have a healthy body. Choosing only one thing to do to reduce your stress is just like only exercising (but not eating right) to create a healthy body. Doing only one thing cannot insure your body's health. You must use a combination of stress reducers to increase your chance of combating stress. This will give you the peace of mind that you can survive through anything.

*"When you change
the way you look at
things the things
you look at change"*

Wayne W. Dyer

# 11

# Bird Flu 911

## *Mistakes You Don't Want To Make*

The greatest mistake I see that people might make is either eliminating beneficial things all together that could help their chance of survival, or doing things that they think are good but hinder their chance of survival. Take a look at the following list. These are common beliefs a person might have. Write down true or false after each statement

## ANSWER TRUE OR FALSE:

1. **I don't need Vitamins since I eat well.**
2. **There is nothing wrong with taking blood thinners.**
    - **Ginger**
    - **Garlic**
    - **Aspirin**
    - **Cumadin**
3. **If I have a cough, cough suppressants are always a good idea.**
4. **Penicillin, Tamiflu or vaccinations will save me.**
5. **Air filters and air purifiers are the same thing.**

6. **One weekend of partying won't hurt me.**
7. **Gathering in large crowds outdoors is okay.**
8. **I can watch things that are scary.**
9. **I'm not sick; therefore, I don't need to watch what I eat.**
10. **I don't need much sleep.**

If you answered *"true"* to any of the above statements, you could be making a big mistake when it comes to the Bird Flu; you need to take another look at the information in this book. Based on these statements I have written the following mistakes a person might make. The mistakes correspond with each false belief.

## 1. ELIMINATING VITAMINS

*I don't need Vitamins since I eat well.*

There are so many things in our society that cause the vitamins we try to get from our food to be inadequate. First of all, most produce is lacking in nutrients.

> *"Thanks to what the chemical agriculture industry calls "artificial manure," supermarket produce appears to be giving today's Americans more salt and less nutrition than generally recognized."*
>
> Dr. Bernard Jensen, Mark Anderson
> Empty Harvest, 1973

Stress affects our emotional state; pollution puts chemical stress on our body. We eat poorly some of the time and in some cases most of the time. All of these things put extra demands on our body. So, even if we were eating right a hundred percent of the time our body loses vitamins just in everyday living.

Some individuals today when they hear that the greatest deaths in 1918 were from the 20-40 year old age group who had the best immune systems, they freak out and say *"to heck with eating right."* As a result some people are foregoing their vitamins and everything else possible to build their immune system. As you probably have guessed, this is a wrong conclusion to make. The people in 1918 happened to be located where the flu started. This age group was at, ground zero, the camp where the flu originated. They were under tremendous amounts of stress; training many hours a day in horrible weather conditions and staying up late at night. The stress from knowing they would soon be deployed to fight a war, as well as the intensive training, resulted in a compromised immune system.

If your decision is to stop taking your vitamins, because those with the best immune system died in 1918, if that is your conclusion, let's go over the contributing factors to these deaths once again. The 20 - 40 year olds were eating mucus causing foods, smoking, staying out late, drinking alcohol and soda (which not only contains sugar but phosphoric acid.) They were under the most stress, because most men in the 20-40 year old group were headed off to war. Stress was the culprit, not a strong immune system that made them more susceptible to disease.

Infants in 1918 had a better survival rate than the 20 - 40 year olds. Why, because breast milk is very alkalizing. Most of the infants were drinking breast milk which is alkaline and does not produce mucus. The elderly survived because they may not have given up their whole grains and raw milk. They also may have developed some immunity during the pandemic thirty years earlier.

Not taking any vitamins maybe a disastrous decision. Most of those who died in 1918 showed signs of severe vitamin C deficiency. This could be what caused the blood vessels to burst and fill their lungs. (See section on *How to Prepare*).

## 2. TAKING A BLOOD THINNER

*There is nothing wrong with taking blood thinners.*

During the Bird Flu, Cumadin or Aspirin may not be the wisest thing to be taking. Remember that the Bird Flu victims often had the capillaries in the lungs burst, allowing their lungs to fill with blood.

Thinner blood may cause the lungs to fill up faster. Consult your doctor to see if taking you off a blood thinner is something you could or should do. Never do it on your own. If he or she thinks you must be on a blood thinner, ask her about substituting your blood thinner with garlic, or even better yet, capsicum. Garlic has blood thinning properties and also antibacterial properties at the same time, so switching from aspirin to garlic will at least give you blood thinning with viral fighting properties.

People with a cold or flu often take garlic to help ward off illness and reduce symptoms. Garlic has great anti-bacterial properties, but remember it also is a blood thinner. If you don't need a blood thinner you may not want to take garlic at all. Taking a blood thinner could cause you to bleed easier. You may be shooting yourself in the foot if you attempt to use garlic, or even ginger for that matter, for Bird Flu.

A great alternative is to take capsicum. Capsicum is a blood thinner but it also has anti-bacterial properties and is great at strengthening blood vessels, while most importantly, at the same time having superior blood coagulating capabilities. Even though Capsicum is a blood thinner, its blood clotting capabilities are far greater. It can stop bleeding quickly and effectively.

I have used capsicum many times to stop bleeding. I swallow a pill or put it directly on a cut. In just minutes the bleeding slows down or stops altogether. To be able to stop bleeding, could be a key factor in creating a Bird Flu resistant body. Capsicum is purchased in bulk or capsule form.

Capsicum can be tolerated easiest if taken in the pill form on a full stomach. It should not be taken on an empty stomach. Capsicum taken on an empty stomach won't kill you, it will most likely give you heart burn. Garlic's anti-bacterial benefit could be great for Bird Flu, since many people died from the flu developing into pneumonia. Don't forget to take it with capsicum to compensate for its blood thinning properties. In combination these two herbs, capsicum and garlic, can have great immune power.

## 3. OVER USING COUGH SUPPRESSANTS

*If you have a cough, cough suppressants are always a good idea.*

Cough suppressants prevent the body from removing mucus from the lungs. If they are taken in the beginning when the lungs are not over stressed, the lungs could start to fill with fluid, leading towards developing pneumonia. Coughing is the body's natural way of expelling mucus and should not be stopped. A person should wait until a doctor prescribes the cough suppressant, which is usually at the recovery phase, towards the end of the illness (when there is no concern about the lungs filling with fluid). Cough Suppressants are often prescribed in the recovery phase, to give the lungs a needed break from coughing; thereby allowing the patient to obtain much needed rest. If Bird Flu is not yet here and you get a cold that involves coughing, you might want to put up with the coughing, because coughing will be good exercise for your lungs. Remember, besides pneumonia, victims of the Bird Flu died because their lungs gave out from coughing too much. Let the doctors decide the right time to take cough suppressants. Leave it up to the experts.

## COUGH SYRUP FOLK REMEDY

**2 slices of a good sized onion**

**1 Cup Honey**

1. **Chop the two slices of onion**
2. **Place honey and onions in a sauce pan**
3. **Simmer until onions appear "see through"**
4. **Strain (or leave the onions in)**
5. **Take one tablespoon as needed**

# 4. DEPENDING ON PENICILLIN, TAMIFLU OR VACCINATIONS

*Penicillin, Tamiflu, or vaccinations will save me.*

What a gamble this is. Will there be enough? Is there time for vaccinations to be produced? Once the Bird Flu mutates, if we are lucky, it will take a minimum of six months to develop a vaccine. Right now vaccinations are produced using chicken eggs. Chicken eggs may be hard to come by during a Bird Flu. Vaccinations cannot be relied upon because there may not be enough to go around. Vaccinations are never one hundred percent effective, so this too is a reason not to depend on them. Rather than rely on a vaccination, prepare your body's immune system to be as strong as it can be, by exercising and eating right.

Remember, penicillin does not work on viruses but on bacteria and even then not all bacteria respond to penicillin. Half of the deaths in 1918 were deaths where pneumonia was not present, so having Penicillin available wouldn't have helped in those cases anyway. What if penicillin is in short supply? If it is, you can always take apple cider vinegar. In D.C. Jarvis, MD's book, *Folk Medicine,* he explains how giving a cow vinegar reduced the amount of bacteria in the milk. I don't know if that will work for preventing a bacterial infection in humans but if there is no penicillin it would be worth a try. What if we don't have an antibiotic or the penicillin is ineffective on the particular bacteria, which develops from the Bird Flu? I'm hitting the apple cider vinegar. Relying on penicillin to be your savior is not a guarantee that you will survive. The influenza virus mutates so rapidly that Tamiflu may not work. Tamiflu may not even be available to all of us. To avoid taking care of yourself, because penicillin and Tamiflu might work is risky business. Why not prepare for the worst and hope for the best? Now that would be more of a guarantee than relying on something that may not work.

If you are turned away from the hospital, another folk remedy option exists: make an onion poultice (herbs applied topically to the skin) and place it on the ill person's chest. Once again, this is not to be used instead of medical attention. Use the following only in the case where no medical attention is available.

## ONION CHEST POULTICE FOLK REMEDY

½ raw onion

1/8 Cup olive oil

hand towel

plastic wrap

tight T-shirt or ace bandage

1. Chop onion
2. Have ill person lie on their back
3. Cover chest with olive oil
4. Spread onions on the chest
5. Cover chest with a towel
6. Wrap the body with plastic wrap
7. Put on a tight T-shirt or ace bandage
8. Wear for 24 hours
9. Repeat as necessary

The onions being in the same family as garlic will help prevent pneumonia and draw out the fluid from the lungs.

## 5. PURCHASING AIR FILTERS INSTEAD OF AIR PURIFIERS

*Air filters and air purifiers are the same thing.*

Air filters move air through the air filter, trapping the particles in the unit. An air purifier changes the air quality, which in turn allows the air to clean itself. Particles combine in the air making them too heavy to stay suspended so they fall to the ground. So what is the difference if the particles are on the ground or in a filter? Air filters cannot move enough air to clean the whole room. The air at the end of the room does not make its way to the filter. Getting around corners is also difficult for air filters. Air purifiers change the chemistry of the air, the room's air quality; therefore, it is more effective as an air cleaner. (See Appendix B for more information on air purifiers)

## 6. OVER CHALLENGING YOUR IMMUNE SYSTEM

*One weekend of partying won't hurt me.*

Some people are bound to think: *"I eat right, exercise and meditate; my body can handle one weekend of partying."* No matter how good your immune system, one weekend of partying can do you in. Not only will you be out in a crowd but alcohol rapidly reduces the body's ability to fight infection. It is worth repeating. In Thomas Appell's book *Never Get Another Cold,* he gives two examples of clients going on a weekend partying spree and then ending up sick, even though they ate alkalizing foods the rest of the time.

Instead of partying now, plan on having a big party for the survivors once the threat of Bird Flu is over and try to have it in June or July, just in case you decide to party prematurely.

## 7. GATHERING IN LARGE CROWDS

*Gathering in large crowds outdoors is okay.*

Gathering in a large group, like in a church or theater, should be avoided during a pandemic. Crowds outdoors can be just as problematic. In Philadelphia the worst part of the pandemic was after the Liberty Loan parade to support the war effort. The parade was well attended and put people in close proximity to one another.

Large crowds indoors or outdoors should be avoided. Even though it would appear being outside would make it easier for you to keep your distance, it is not. At a sports game, even if you were to sit a bleacher row away from anyone, in just getting to your seat you will come in close contact with others. At a sports game crowds stand close to each other to purchase tickets or refreshments. When the game ends everyone leaves at the same time, bunching up at the exits. A crowd is a crowd indoors or out.

## 8. SCARY THINGS DON'T BOTHER ME

*I can watch things that are scary.*

Your viewing of the news repeatedly during an emergency, or watching a scary movie, will start the fight or flight response in your body. Sugar will be released into your blood stream in preparation to fight or run. If you do not run, you have just made your blood stream very acidic. If someone in the household is sick you have just set yourself up for illness. Make sure if you are going to watch something that scares you that you plan on how you are going to get your body to calm down. Will you exercise, drink chamomile tea, take extra B vitamins or use Bach Flower Rescue remedy? Have a plan. Life will be scary enough; don't add to it during a pandemic.

## 9. WAITING TO EAT RIGHT

*I'm not sick; therefore, I don't need to watch what I eat.*

You need to start now. The Bird Flu is rather quick to take hold. You won't have time to go shopping later. The time just won't be there to set up your home for a fail safe environment, like Dr. Phil suggests when you are trying to eat right. Set up your home, NOW! Get used to different eating habits, NOW! It is easier to do when you are not under a lot of stress.

When someone in the house is sick, watch what you eat. Don't sit down to a big steak dinner with mash potatoes and gravy. Choose instead to eat a salad for dinner and a fruit smoothie for breakfast. Choose to drink liquid Chlorophyll instead of coffee. Making better food choices is most important, if someone is sick in the house. Keeping others in the household from getting sick will reduce exposure. Besides, if you manage to stay well during a family member's illness, your body will be creating antibodies, which will protect you from getting the flu.

When we are stressed our food choices are usually compromised. We should set up our home to be a fail safe environment. This will make it easier to make better choices.

## 10. NOT GETTING ENOUGH SLEEP

*I don't need much sleep.*

Even if you feel you normally only require six hours of sleep, try and get more. If you just can't sleep that long, use the extra time to do deep breathing exercises or to meditate. Your body will still be getting more rest and have an easier time supporting your immune system.

You don't want to have sleep deprived stress. Just don't stay up late! It will lower your immune system, so don't do it!

# 12

# If Your City Is Unprepared For Bird Flu, What To Do!

## *Knowing what to do, if your city is not providing you with information will give you peace of mind*

As a Civil Engineer, I have worked with several different city planning departments. I have noticed that some cities are more organized than others. In 1918 in Philadelphia the wealthy ended up taking over control of the city when the city's infrastructure broke down. They were the ones that had the power in the community. During a pandemic there may be a shift in the powers that be, order will need to be maintained. I am including the following to give you some idea as to what needs to be done, if your city falls short.

The following section can be quite scary to think about. Be warned, it may freak you out. This may be tough to take by some individuals but it must be said. No one else wants to admit that this can happen. I am here to tell you that it can and you will want to be prepared. When the Bird Flu hit and overwhelmed the medical system in 1918, a horrible disturbing situation resulted. Many dead were left without the respect of a proper burial. (Just like the horrible images we saw with the Katrina victims in 2005). In 1918 there was no one willing to come and take the bodies to their final resting place. Families would leave the body in the room where the person died, close the door, and stuff rags under the door to try and keep out the odor of the decomposing body. Some bodies were put on porches or in back yards. Some families were desperate enough to take the body to a cemetery themselves, digging a grave and burying their own dead.

Some relatives left their homes after a family member passed away. They were too afraid to touch the body or move it in any way for fear of getting the flu.

In an emergency situation, you just may have to deal with a family member that has passed and I want to offer some guidance in what you can do. If you follow my advice, it may make it more appealing to workers to retrieve your loved one and put their body in a respectable place. It will also help identify your loved one in case bodies are buried in mass graves as was the case in 1918. Having your loved one properly wrapped and identified will make finding their body in a mass grave easier. You may want to later, when the resources are available, bury your loved one properly. No one wants to think about it but as horrible as it is to imagine, we just may have to take extreme measures to bury our dead.

If you have a queasy stomach you may want to skip this section but make sure you keep this book as a reference.

Why even talk about dead bodies? Funeral homes in a small town are set up to handle on average of 5-10 bodies at a time max. When a national disaster hits, the usual protocol is that the county or state medical examiners take over and runs the show. Now what do you do if all the cities in a state are having an emergency at the same time. Then what?

A city can do many things now to prepare for the Bird Flu (See further details in Appendix C, City Preparedness Planning).

The City of Philadelphia was not prepared. In Philadelphia the wealthy families took over where the city was lacking leadership. You may have to be the leader that helps your city make it through. The City Preparedness Plan will guide you as to what needs to be done to help your city function.

## IF SOMEONE IN YOUR HOUSEHOLD TAKES ILL

1. Take the person to the nearest hospital and notify your street leader

2. If hospital is full, keep ill person at home.

## DEATH IN THE HOUSEHOLD - WHAT TO DO?

1. *Wear gloves while you wrap the body in a sheet; then place it in a body bag. If a body bag is not available, wrap body with plastic tablecloth (or shower curtain) using duct tape to securely fasten plastic around body. Some body fluids may leak so make sure you use plenty of duct tape.*

2. *Identify deceased with a note written in permanent ink or pencil.*

3. *Place identification note into plastic sandwich bag, duct tape it to the body and write identification information directly onto the plastic tablecloth with a permanent marker.*
   *Include name, sex, birth date and date of death.*

   ***Example: Jon Smith, Male, birth (month/ day/ year), death (month/ day/ year)***

4. *If you are unable to contact officials, move body to curb*

5. *Clean room, using apple cider vinegar and water*

6. *Wash sheets and bedding in hot water. If hot water is not available, due to loss of electricity, use metal trashcan to burn sheets*

7. *Air out room and mattress. Putting mattress in the sun will help.*

Organize your neighbors. Hand out this form before the first citizen takes ill. Each street / apartment building should implement a Street Leader position. They should elect or appoint a person to be the Street Leader and alternate Street Leader. This person(s), since you may need an alternate in case the leader becomes ill, will conduct a census of homes on the street, including all the family members living in each home as well as occupations.

Use the flag color system below to notify others of what is happening in your household.

## BIRD FLU HOME FLAG SYSTEM

**White Flag** - means all is clear, no one is sick

**Red flag** - means illness is in the home

**Black flag** - indicates a death has taken place.

# 13

# Preventing A Break In Your Medical Care

## *Knowing how to take over your medical care even if you are taking medications could save your life*

Why should you be concerned about the hospital's ability to provide care? Plain and simple, hospitals have streamlined to lower costs. We have fewer beds per capita today than we did in the sixties. No longer is there a lot of excess capacity built into the system. Less capacity means fewer extra beds, which in turn means hospitals will fill up faster during a pandemic and the healthcare system will become overwhelmed quicker. This is why having this book on hand, readily available, is more important than ever.

Remember that doctors and nurses are people too! They have families and loved ones to care for, as well as patients. I see doctors, nurses and all hospital staff being in great demand.

The American Red Cross came to the aid of many people in 1918 but they too often fell short of medical personnel. Trying to mount a massive relief effort, as I'm sure the Red Cross will do, could be an overwhelming task. By making a donation now to the Red Cross will help the Red Cross stock up on supplies. The better prepared they are the better off we will be.

As a potential patient you need to do what you can now to make medical personnel's life easier. Ask questions now, while your doctor is not stressed and has plenty of time to prepare an answer, as to how you personally should prepare for the Bird Flu.

Ask any and all questions you can think of regarding your current medical care. Below are some of the questions you might want to ask your doctor now!

## WHAT TO ASK YOUR DOCTOR NOW, BEFORE THE BIRD FLU IS A THREAT!

1. What protocol should I follow, if Bird Flu does occur?
    a. How often should I wash my hands?
    b. When should I wear a mask?
    c. Would it be a good idea to tape to the refrigerator a list of medications I am currently taking?

2. What foods, herbs or vitamins might have a negative affect with my medication?

3. How should I treat an ill person in my home?

4. How will I know when I should seek medical attention?

5. What procedure should I follow if I cannot get into a hospital? (This is very important especially if you are already being treated for a medical condition.)

6. How will my current condition be affected or complicated by the Bird Flu?

7. What should I do if I cannot obtain my medication?

8. Will my medication cause:
    a. Thinning of the blood
    b. Lower immune response
    c. Cause constipation?
    d. If so, are there any alternatives?

## Preventing A Break In Your Medical Care

The time to get with your doctor to develop a plan is now! After reading the first chapter you should be aware that waiting to ask is not an option. There are many foods, herbs and vitamins that when combined with medication could produce complications. Before you decide what you are going to do for the Bird Flu discuss your plan with your doctor. Have them review your plan now before the Bird Flu hits.

*Medical personnel and their families may want to refer to Appendix D. This section will give the medical person some things to think about.*

*"A danger foreseen*
*is half avoided."*

Thomas Fuller

# 14

# How To Survive!

## *Bird Flu has arrived, now what should you do?*

The first thing you will need to learn is to recognize the symptoms associated with the Bird Flu. At first the symptoms are very similar to normal seasonal flu symptoms: body aches, fever, sore throat, and coughing. Then the symptoms get worse. Some websites and books like mine have given the symptoms of the Bird Flu, however from their definition it looks like the seasonal flu and the Bird Flu have the same symptoms. It seems like it is not going to be that bad. The books neglect to differentiate the seasonal flu from the Bird Flu. The seasonal flu symptoms are only the beginning symptoms of the Bird Flu.

Let's take it one step further, what makes the Bird Flu different from the seasonal flu? There are three more dramatic symptoms not found in the seasonal flu associated with the Bird Flu. These extra symptoms are found in Kolata's, Crosby's and Barry's books. When we keep these symptoms in mind we can plan ahead to prevent them before they even happen. You need more than the facts and symptoms of the less severe seasonal flu. Having all the facts would help you to make better choices for you and your family.

## Symptoms

**Body aches** - an infected person will develop joint pain. It will be hard for them to get comfortable.

**Fever** - As the body is trying to fight off the invasion, the immune system is stimulated by a rise in temperature. Bacteria cannot live in elevated temperatures; therefore, the fever is a good thing. The ill person may experience times of delirium, or not in their right state of mind. This state can last three or more days after the fever breaks.

**Coughing** - the ill person will begin to have coughing fits and sometimes will continually cough. The coughing may be unproductive.

**Sore Throat** - sore throats are a common symptom of the Bird Flu; however they are not always present.

**Blood will discharge** from the nose, ears, and eye sockets - This will happen as the disease progresses.

**Skin will start to turn blue** - This is because the ill person cannot get enough oxygen. Blood in the body is blue when there is no oxygen. The skin will start with just patches of blue, increasing the patch sizes until the skin is all or mostly blue.

**Labored breathing** - breathing will become more and more difficult.

## WHAT TO DO?

### Possible at Home Treatments:

I have chosen to include a list of symptoms and alternatives in this book, since there may be a time that you cannot get into the hospital. This is not medical advice and should not be substituted for medical attention; it is in case there is none available. Following my advice will be at your own risk; however, based on my research and with the help of Jack Ritchason's, *Little Herb Encyclopedia*, you at least can help yourself, if there is no other advice and treatment available.

**Body aches** - Magnesium has been known to relax the muscles. Coral Calcium is for the acidic condition in the body that may be attributing to the body aches.

**Fever** - If fever is mild the use of a far-inferred sauna to help elevate the temperature to 104 degrees Fahrenheit to prevent bacterial growth, which may prevent a secondary bacterial infection. Since heat has been known to kill viruses and bacteria, a fever will help to stimulate the immune system and prevent bacterial growth. Cold compresses can be used to reduce fevers over 104 degrees Fahrenheit. Elevated fevers above 104 degrees Fahrenheit have been known to cause an ill person to become incoherent or cause delirium. So, understand a person with an elevated fever may make unrealistic demands. An ill person with a fever should be kept hydrated (See the electrolyte folk remedy).

**Coughing** - Prepare and use the folk remedy cough syrup described in this book. The cough syrup will not suppress the cough, but break up the mucus and allow the mucus to be expelled easier. The onion poultice can be applied, if the cough is not responding to the cough syrup.

**Sore Throat** - zinc lozenges help with sore throats. Brew up some sore throat tea (See recipe below).

**Blood will discharge** from nose, ears and eye sockets – Capsicum, vitamin C and Calcium will help prevent this from happening and should be started at the first signs of illness. If an ill person has reached this stage, increase the amount of vitamin C,

Capsicum and Calcium, making sure to give it with food, to prevent heartburn. The ill person's body will require a lot of vitamin C. Capsicum will help stop any bleeding and since the *b. influenza bacteria* needs blood to reproduce, anything you use to prevent bleeding could help.

**Skin will start to turn blue** - Liquid Chlorophyll will help with iron absorption and thereby help with oxygen uptake. Getting any and all mucus out will help (refer to onion poultice and cough syrup folk remedies).

**Labored breathing** – You should have attempted to bring the ill to the hospital way before this happens, but if you were turned away, try to get the ill person outside for fresh air. If breathing becomes labored, try to use the onion poultice described in this book. By addressing all of the symptoms hopefully labored breathing will lessen too.

## SORE THROAT TEA FOLK REMEDY

**1 cup water**

**1 teaspoon Slippery Elm Bark herb**

**1 packet Stevia**

**1 wedge of lemon, if available**

1. **Boil water in a sauce pan**
2. **Remove from heat**
3. **Add herb**
4. **Let it seep or set for 20 minutes**
5. **Strain**
6. **Add Stevia and lemon**
7. **Drink warm, not hot!**

## MAINTAIN CAUTION!

In 1918 after a person was feeling better, two weeks or longer, after their recovery, they became ill again. A person who seemed to have recovered would relapse, become seriously ill with pneumonia, a secondary bacterial infection. This secondary infection often led to death.

It is a good idea to spend one month, if not more, recovering.

*“The wise man avoids evil
by anticipating it.”*

Publilius Syrus

# 15

# Food Storage And Stocking Up

## *How to tell what you have and what you need*

Some people say that stocking our homes in case a Bird Flu should ever arise is over-doing it or being fearful. To me it just makes common sense. We never know when a disaster is going to hit and being prepared for the worst is never a bad thing. We saw with Katrina what not heeding a warning can do. Throughout history we know famine and disasters have struck. So rather than sticking your head in the sand, why not choose to be prepared?

## Steps to getting prepared

In order to be prepared we need to follow some simple steps. I have found with my own family it took one month to sort through what I have, what I need to be prepared and buy what I was missing. If these steps are too much for you to handle, see pg 179, Storage System. The Storage System has worksheets and a CD to help you with a step by step guide in how to determine what you need.

### 1. Inventory

First you must inventory what you have. Use the following *Disaster Preparation Check List* on page 127 to determine what you have and make a list of what you are missing.

## 2. Date and mark all consumables

Go around your house with a permanent marker and date all your consumables right on the package. Make a fill line across the bottle or box to measure how much is presently in the package or product. For example, on my cereal box I will write today's date and a straight line 1/3 of the way down the package (because the box was open and partially used). The next time I open a box I will compare my line with what is actually inside the new box. This will give me an idea of how much I have used.

If this is too difficult, to make it easier: on the week you begin your *"information gathering week"* only use new boxes of products; how much you use will be easier to see and determine. Since most products are not filled to the top, be sure to mark a fill line. This line will be used to tell you where you began and where you ended up.

## 3. Determine how much you use

To do this take a week to gather data. Your *Information Gathering Week* will start and end on a Saturday. When you begin write down how much you have of each item. Do this right on the box of cereal with a permanent marker. Write *"½ box of cereal"*; on a bottle of shampoo, write *"1/3 bottle of shampoo."* Write dates on all items. Do this with various items throughout your house. Write the numbers 1,2,3,4 on the side of each roll of toilet paper. At the end of the week whichever number you ended on will tell you how much you used. If you have a half of a roll of number three left, then you used 2 ½ rolls for that week.

## 4. Record or save packages you have consumed during your *"Information Gathering Week"*

Keep track of what you consume for one week. Don't throw out your packages. Save all bottles and packages for one week in a box.

This will make it easier for you to determine how much you use without having to write everything down as you use it. At the end of the week empty the box and record what your family has consumed. After a week, two of the things I determined that I used were toilet paper and shampoo, among other things. I recorded that I used two (2) and a half rolls of toilet paper and an eighth of a bottle of shampoo. From there you have a good idea of how much toilet paper you will need. You can now figure out how much you would need for a month or six months. To find out how much exactly you would require for six months I have developed a storage system (See Appendix E). This system contains math formulas for figuring out your needs. If you are not inclined to do the math, check out our website. You can send your data to us (www.escapethebirdflu.com) and for a small charge we will figure it out for you.

## Disaster Preparation Check List

The following is a Disaster Check List. It will guide you in what to have in stock. It is not a complete list, since I am finding things all the time to add to it. I suggest you use it as a guide when deciding your family's needs.

Why is it more important today to prepare for a disaster? Our grocery stores no longer have a warehouse in the back filled with food. Today stores supply their store on a more daily or weekly supply system, meaning that when product comes in, it is immediately put on the shelves and does not spend much time in the receiving part of the store. Therefore, if a fluctuation occurs in the trucking system, our store shelves may become bare. In Florida we noticed right away that the ports in New Orleans had been hit by a major hurricane (Katrina). Bananas and several other fruits were missing from our shelves for weeks. If the disaster had been more widespread, what else would we have found missing from our shelves?

Your needs will be different from mine but you may want to consider creating a list for your own family, using mine as a guide.

Remember, transportation will be greatly affected in the event of the Bird Flu. This interruption in food supply and material goods could last six months to two years before it returns to normal. With so many people out sick, we may not have pilots, mechanics, truckers, factory workers, harvesters, and farmers, able to keep and deliver our supplies. In the event of a Bird Flu we need to have our pantry and home ready to be self- sufficient in order to withstand a long term disaster.

After each list, a short explanation will follow. I will explain what the items are used for and how to use them. A list is no good unless you know what to do with the things on the list.

## LINENS

Washcloths
Towels
Sheets
Hand towels
Plastic mattress cover
Plastic tablecloth or shower curtain

You will need at least two sets of linen for each bed, two towels and washcloths per person; this way, one set can be washed while the other is being used. If you cover the mattress with a plastic tablecloth or plastic mattress cover, it will help keep the bed healthy in the event of an illness or death.

## KITCHEN ITEMS

Sponge
Hand towels
Cast Iron Pots and Pans

## KITCHEN ITEMS Continued

- Can Opener
- Dish Soap
- Utensils
  - Long handled utensils
  - Spoons
  - Forks
  - Ladle
  - Spatula
- Natural Cleaners
- Plastic utensils
- Paper plates
- Paper towels
- Plastic wrap (for poultice)
- Plastic sandwich bags
  (for body identification information)

Think of your kitchen and what you need to run it. Make sure you have the things you need. Have enough dish soap on hand to last at least a year to a year and a half. In 1918 the Bird Flu took that long to run its course. Long handled utensils will come in handy if you have to cook over a gas stove or fire. In case the power is shut off, paper towels can be used to wash the dishes, and for cleaning. If you are washing dishes without power you will need to sterilize the silverware with boiling water, or use plastic utensils you can throw away. Natural cleansers, such as Apple Cider Vinegar, mixed with water, or baking soda, are less of a challenge to your immune system.

## CLOTHING

Bras
Gloves
Jackets
Jeans
Socks
Durable shoes
Sewing Kit
Shirts (long and short sleeves)
Shorts
Undies
Long underwear

Think of everything you need to wear in both the winter and summer. A two week supply of clothing with an outfit for everyday should be enough; however, if someone in your family has an illness, they may need to change more frequently. You should have at least 14 pairs of socks and undies for each person. Make sure you have clothing, shoes and jackets, a size up (undies too), for your growing child(ren). A sewing kit will come in handy when trying to keep clothing functioning and wearable. During a pandemic you may lose weight and will need some way of doing alterations.

## FOODS

7- Day Meal Plan
Baking Soda (electrolyte home remedy)
Beans
Brewer's Yeast (for popcorn flavoring and Biotin)
Brown sugar
Brown Rice (Biotin and electrolyte home remedy)
Canned fruits & Vegetables
Canned Soup (or dry soups)
Crackers

Dried Fruit and Vegetables
Dried apples/banana
Dried Potatoes
Dried Peas and carrots
Fresh Fruits
Grains (whole)
Honey (for cough syrup)
Jelly
Juice (bottled or canned)
Nuts
Oatmeal (Biotin)
Olive oil (for poultice)
Peanut Butter (Biotin) made without sugar
Popcorn
Powdered Eggs
Powdered Milk
Powdered Butter
Salt
Seasoning (favorite spices)
Seeds
Shelf milk – (Soy, almond, rice)
Vegetables (especially Onions for a poultice)
Vinegar (apple cider)
Water

If the power goes out, your frig will be without electricity so stock your pantry with foods that do not require refrigeration. Put together at least seven recipes for dinner, including soups, pancakes, beans and rice.

Remember, biotin is a nutrient used in glucose metabolism and pH balancing. Whole grains can be soaked in water with dried fruit overnight and eaten in the morning for breakfast. Oatmeal could be another alternative. Beans, nuts and seeds will provide a good source of protein. Look for shelf milk in your grocery store, it has a long shelf life and can be kept in your pantry.

When a person is sick with the Bird Flu, he or she should stay away from mucus causing foods such as dairy and wheat products, if available, stick to non-milk based soups and fresh fruits and vegetables. In 1918, the lungs of those who died contained large amounts of fluids, some of which was mucus. Limiting mucus producing foods could help reduce the amount of fluid entering the lungs.

Make sure you have fresh onions on hand to make a poultice and cough syrup, along with Lemons; they can be used in the electrolyte formula and sore throat tea. Make sure when considering fresh fruits and vegetables to include the ones from the Alkalizing foods list found in section two in the chapter titled "*How to Prepare.*" Have plenty of seeds for growing edible sprouts. Sprouting seeds to make sprouts for eating are different than seeds for sprouting to grow plants in the ground. (See *Miscellaneous* section for more information.)

## BABY

Baby Shampoo
Baby Food Grinder
Bibs
Clothing (next two to four sizes up)
Diaper cream
Diapers (cloth, a couple of sizes)
Lavender Essential Oil
Toy (birthday gift)
Vinegar (apple cider)
Wipes (cloth) 50 per child

Since adults can also use baby shampoo, only stock baby shampoo. The baby food grinder is for making baby food. We want to make sure someone without teeth will be able to eat. Clothing for your child is a must. Because a lot of clothing and toys are made in China, and ships may be quarantined, you will need a supply of several outfits for your growing child. Don't forget to include jackets, socks, shoes, and a toy for a birthday or two. The child may not remember his/her birthday in a time of a crisis, but a celebration will help the whole family's mood. Store enough gifts for two years. It is not necessary to buy a lot of gifts; a single gift per child would be greatly appreciated in a time of distress.

Diapers should be obtained in several sizes, since your child will be growing. Cloth diapers come in a variety of types; the best ones I've found are purchased on the web and are made by stay at home moms. These diapers are adjustable, with elastic backs and legs and use snaps instead of pins for fastening. You may want to buy some just in case the disposable ones are not available. Don't forget the plastic pants, since cloth diapers are not waterproof. Have plenty of rags that can be used for wipes or make sure you have extra paper towels on hand in case your wipe supply runs low.

Remember to have enough supplies for 12-18 months. If you plan to only stock ready-made wipes, make sure you cycle them out or they can mold. Cloth wipes can be made from rags and wet with the following recipe:

## BABY WIPE RECIPE

**1/4 Cup Apple Cider Vinegar**

**2 ½ Cup Water**

**2-3 drops of Lavender oil**

**Mix together and pour over rags (instant wipes)**

Lavender oil can be purchased from a company online called "*Frontier*." Several drops of lavender oil in a bath can calm an upset child or infant.

## MISCELLANEOUS

Auto cell phone charger
Ax or Hatchet
Batteries
Bucket
Candles
Duct tape (to secure bodies)
Flashlight
Food saver
Lantern / candles
Manual can opener
Mop and an extra mop head or two
Permanent Marker (body identification)
Pet food and supplies
Phone with a cord and cell phone
Plastic Tablecloth or shower curtain (for body bag)
Prescriptions
Radio with Batteries
Rope
Scissors
Seeds
Sewing kit
Soaps and Cleansers
Sprouter (or quart size glass jar and lid) for sprouting seeds
Square Foot Gardening Book, by Mel Bartholomew
Tissue

Scissors are for cutting duct tape and rope. Ax or Hatchet is for cutting and splitting wood. Having a couple of buckets on hand, in case a person in your home is throwing up: one bucket can be used to hold the mop and water to clean up if they miss the other bucket. Plastic tablecloths can be put on the bed, as well as under the bucket beside the bed. Plastic tablecloth or plastic shower curtains can also be used as a body bag in the event a coroner is not available.

In case the electricity goes off, your radio, flashlight, candles or lantern can be used to provide light. A cell phone will work for a limited amount of time without electricity to charge it; however, a phone with a cord attached from the handset to the phone base will work without electricity. Having both phones on hand is a good idea. If food is in short supply, vegetable and fruit seeds can be used to create a garden.

Keep seeds in a glass jar in your fridge until ready to use. Do not mix up seeds for sprouting and seeds for planting. Seeds meant for planting often have chemicals added to aid in their sprouting. You will not want to eat sprouts made from these seeds; however, eating the vegetable or fruit they produce is perfectly fine, but to put them on a salad is not recommended. Having sprouts will assure that you will have produce during the winter months, since salad sprouts can be grown in the house in a glass jar. All you do is poke holes in the top, put some seeds in, add water and drain out through the holes daily; the sprouts will sprout in a couple of days.

The *New Square Foot Gardening* book, by Mel Bartholomew, will allow you to grow a lot of food in a small area. I was surprised at how well Mel's system works. My garden this year was one third the size it was before and my yield was much greater. The neat thing about square foot gardening is that it can be done anywhere, even from city roof tops, to balconies, to your back yard.

## LARGE ITEMS

Air purifier
Generator
Humidifier
Metal trash can
Portable gas heater
Portable Toilet
Stove or BBQ grill (gas or wood)
Water Barrels
Water purification system
Wood (if you have a fire place)

You can use a portable stove or BBQ grill for cooking if power is not available. The metal trashcan becomes a make-shift grill when placing an oven rack on top. Holes may need to be put on the side near the bottom of the trashcan to ventilate the fire. Use extreme caution when using a make shift grill. Cooking outside will be a lot different than cooking on a stove since you cannot set the temperature. Since trash collection may not be available, you might want to have two trashcans, one to burn your trash in and the other for cooking. A portable gas heater is necessary in the winter months, if the electricity is turned off. If you don't have a gas heater make sure you have long underwear.

Generator caution: **DO NOT** turn your generator on in the house. It **MUST** be outside. Generators produce a deadly fume called carbon dioxide, which can kill everyone in the house if you run the generator inside.

Even if you have water it may not contain the chemicals required to purify it, so a water purification system is a must. The flu virus does not flourish in humidity. This is why in the summer we have fewer incidences of the flu than we have in the winter. The heating of your home in the winter dries out the air. A humidifier can replace the lost humidity due to the heating of the home. Use water barrels to collect rainwater from your roof. This water can be used to flush your toilets or water a garden. A portable toilet is useful when a person is sick. The ill person will not need to move as far to use the toilet.

## FIRST AID KIT

- Bach flower remedy
- Band-Aids
- Bug spray
- A cut closing gel
- Disinfectant
- Disposable gloves
- Essential Oils
    - Eucalyptus
    - Camphor
    - Ti fu
    - Breath Free
- First aid tape
- Gauze
- Hydrogen Peroxide
- Iodine
- N95 or N100 masks
- Neosporin
- Rubbing alcohol
- Soap
- Thermometer
- Homeopathic medicine
    - Hypericum
    - Ledum
    - Arnicare
    - Ignatia

If the hospitals are over loaded you may have to take care of the simpler things yourself. Make sure you have all sizes of Band-Aids (large, small, finger and the butterfly type). Gauze and tape can be used for larger problems. Antiseptic, hydrogen peroxide and rubbing alcohol will also be good to have on hand. A first aid book would come in handy too. Think of every conceivable injury you might have and might need for that injury.

The homeopathic medicine Hypericum and Ledum are commonly used for puncture wounds. In the event that you are unable to get a tetanus shot these will come in handy. Ignatia is a homeopathic treatment for grief. Bach flower remedy is commonly used for stress. If the electrical power is shut off in the summer, bug sprays may be necessary. The bug sprays with deet are very toxic and lower the immune system. Try to find natural alternatives to help keep your immune system healthy. Many natural bug sprays are made from Essential Oils, and these sprays are less damaging to the immune system. The Essential Oils listed above help when a person is having trouble breathing, such as the respiratory problems caused by the Bird Flu.

## PERSONAL ITEMS

Creme rinse
Deodorant
Eye contact solution
Feminine products
Floss
Medications
Mouth wash
Prescriptions
Razor blades
Shampoo
Shaving cream
Toilet Paper
Tooth Paste
Tooth Brushes (several)

Have enough feminine products for 12-18 periods per menstruating women in the household. The *Glad Rags* Company makes cloth feminine pads, which can be found in most health food stores. For other conditions you might have, not related to Bird Flu, check with your doctor for the supply of prescriptions or medications you should have on hand.

## SUPPLEMENTS

Bifidophilus
Bulk Slippery Elm Bark
Calcium
Capsicum
Cherry Bark
Echinacea/Goldenseal
Fish Oils
Horehound
Mullein
Multi-Vitamin
Vitamin C
Vitamin B
Zinc

Don't forget in 1918 those who died had shown signs of scurvy, a vitamin C deficiency. Vitamin C and calcium strengthens capillaries, which are one of the things that burst in the lungs causing them to fill up with fluid. Calcium alkalizes the body making it un-virus friendly. Fish oils have vitamin D which aids in the absorption of calcium. The next most important thing to have on hand is capsicum. Remember capsicum will stop hemorrhaging. Garlic is a blood thinner and should not be taken without capsicum. You are bound to be under stress; Vitamin B is for the stress of watching a lot of people dying all around you. Bifidophilus produce vitamin K which aids in blood clotting. A good multi-vitamin will help keep the body healthy. Echinacea and Goldenseal aid the immune system while Mullein, Cherry bark, and Horehound work on controlling mucus.

## IF YOU LEAVE YOUR HOME

Take the above as well as:

- Cash
- Family Photos
- Important Papers
  - Driver's license
  - Insurance
  - Marriage License
  - Will
  - Charge card information
  - Mortgage
  - Birth Certificates
  - Social Security Card
  - Stocks / Bonds
- Pillows
- Sleeping Bags
- Tarp and/or Tent

# 16

# Bulk Food Home Storage Made Easy

## *Storing In bulk will take up less room in your home*

So far you have learned what you need and how much you should store. Storing six months worth of cereal can over time limit your storage space. Another way you can store food is in bulk. The following is a guide in how to store food in bulk. Storing in bulk may require extra skills, like learning how to make flour and cooking from a recipe, to make bulk storage successful. If this is not for you, than you can just stick to the non-bulk way of storing food. An advantage to using bulk foods is that it has less chance of becoming infested with bugs or other unwanted pests. Also bulk foods can be stored in a basement with ease, leaving more room in your cupboards.

Store high quality products away from moisture and light. Only store the foods you plan to eat on a regular basis. Rotate stored food now instead of hoarding it. Keeping your stock rotated will guarantee you will have food stored for years to come.

Foods will store for different lengths of time, depending on how they are stored. Nuts and seeds store longer in the freezer. Grains will keep longest if nitrogen packed and the least if stored in regular containers. Oils containing antioxidants will last longer than other oils. Rotate can goods to lengthen storage time and prevent settling. Do not eat anything that contains mold. The only exception is cheese, in which the mold can be cut off and discarded. Believe it or not foods that contain bugs could be okay to eat.

In order for you to be able to use grains, in a variety of ways, you will need to purchase a grain mill and learn how to process the grains into flour. Vita mix is the easiest one to work with. It will not only process grains but also can be used as a kitchen blender. A non-electric grain mill would also be handy if the electricity is out. If you do not have a mill but for some reason have the grains, you can soak the grains in water overnight to soften and make them edible. You can then strain the grains, or just drink the grain water, add a little sweetener, dried fruit, nuts and you now have a meal.

# Eat, Rotate, Replace (ERR)

## DON'T HOARD

Eat

Rotate

Replace

## WHERE TO STORE

- **Away from heat and humidity**
- **In a clean dry place**
- **In a place where temperature is less than eighty-three degrees**
- **Cool corner of a dry basement**
- **Closet on the north side of the house**
- **Along an inside wall in summer**
- **Along an outside wall in winter**

## NO-NO'S

- **Do not** store directly on concrete floor
- **Do not** store near bathroom
- **Do not** use pesticides in food storage area
- **Do not** have buckets touching

On the next few pages you will find storage charts. The first chart shows how much to store for one person for six months. This chart is followed by a spoilage chart, which will help you tell if your stored food is edible or spoiled.

## HOW MUCH TO STORE FOR 6 MONTHS PER GROWN ADULT

| | |
|---|---|
| Baking soda | 2 lbs |
| Beans | 15 lbs |
| Can fruit | 32 lbs |
| Can vegetables | 32 lbs |
| Dried fruit | 20 #10 cans |
| Dried vegetables | 20 #10 cans |
| Dried Milk | 40 lbs |
| Dry yeast | ½ lb |
| Drains | 100 lbs |
| Honey | 2 gal |
| Nuts | 5 lbs |
| Oil | 15 lbs |
| Pasta | 5 lbs |
| Rice | 100 lbs |
| Salt | 2 lbs |
| Drinking Water | 140-200 gal |

| Stored Product | Storage Time | Spoiled if ... | Not Spoiled if.... |
|---|---|---|---|
| Can Goods | 2-5 years | Bulging or bent cans | |
| Canned Meats | 4-5 years | Bulging or bent cans | |
| Canned Vegetables | 3-4 years | Bulging or bent cans | |
| Canned Fruit | 2-3 years | Bulging or bent cans | |
| Canned legumes | 4-5 years | Bulging or bent cans | |
| Dried Fruit | 1 year | Moldy | Soggy or infested |
| Dried vegetables | 1 year | Moldy | Soggy or infested |
| Evaporated Milk | 12 months | Color or Odor change | |
| Grains | 2-20 years | Moldy | Infested |
| Honey | several years | | Crystallized |
| Mayonnaise | few months | Color or Odor change | |
| Non-citrus fruit juice | 1 year | Bulging or bent cans | |
| Nut butters | 6 months | Odor change | separation of oil |
| Nuts in the shell | 1-2 years | Moldy | |

| Stored Product | Storage Time | Spoiled if ... | Not Spoiled if.... |
|---|---|---|---|
| Olive Oil | 6-8 months | Odor rancid smell not sweet | |
| Pasta | 1-2 years | Disintegrated or moldy | |
| Powered Milk | 2-3 years | Color or Odor change | Caking |
| Salt | almost indefinitely | | May yellow |
| Seeds | 1-2 years | Moldy | |
| Sesame oil | 6-8 months | Odor change | |
| Vinegar (Apple Cider) | several years | Cloudy or sediment | |
| Water | 1 mo -2 yrs | Moldy | Off taste |
| White sugar | several years | | |
| Yeast | 2-3 years | | |

## HOW TO RECLAIM YOUR FOOD

There is a good chance that some of us will find Insects have taken over our home storage. Most insects are a good source of protein and are not poisonous. Remember this book is for worst case scenarios. I hope you never have to reclaim your food, but just in case, this is how it is done:

Not all items will have bugs in them. Some items like water, salt and honey just need a little help to make them fresh again.

**Grains, pastas, dried fruits and vegetables** - if infested with bugs, but not moldy, place in a shallow pan in the oven at 150 degrees for 20 minutes, or freeze for several days.

**Water**, if it becomes stale, pour it from one container to another, back and forth, until stale flavor is gone. Contaminated water can be boiled for 20 minutes.

**Honey,** if crystallized, heat container with lid open until crystals become liquid.

**Salt**, if caked, heat in oven (on low) to dry out

## STORAGE CHECK LIST

- ✓ Storage area location - basement or north side of the house
- ✓ Food grade *"Diatomaceous Earth"* on floor to keep bugs out
- ✓ Food containers stored off the floor
- ✓ No moisture in storage area
- ✓ Stored away from light

It is my hope that you have found the information contained in this book helpful. I hope it has given you some useful tools in the event of a pandemic. I am sure I have missed some things in my desperate attempt to get this out before the next flu season. If you signup for updates on my website **www.escapethebirdflu.com,** I will keep you posted on new information as it comes available.

**May God bless us all in the times that lie ahead!**

*"Knowledge without wisdom*
*is like a library*
*with its doors locked."*

Brendanne Phillips

## Appendix A

# The Experts And The Factors Surrounding The Bird Flu

The following will give you a basic understanding of what happens during a pandemic. Understanding the background will make it easier to understand the ways you can help your body and family to be prepared to fight the Bird Flu. You will understand more fully why stress and exposure are key elements in preventing the Bird Flu. Both of these elements need to be addressed in order to stay healthy. To illustrate the roles of these elements I will be discussing four doctors. These doctors' combined works will allow you to see how the Bird Flu spreads among a population. Combined, their work can give us insights where alone their ideas are not fully understood.

## THE DOCTORS

1. **Hans Selye** - Known for his work relating to stress and illness.
2. **Richard Shope** - Tried to explain the Bird Flu of 1918 with experiments involving pigs.
3. **Robert Koch** - Developed Koch's Postulates, or the Germ Theory.
4. **Max Von Pettenkofer** - Rivaled Koch's theory, believing more than just the pathogen (germ or virus) is responsible for the disease.

If you were to read Hans Selye's work, you would understand that there is a connection between stress and disease. He is widely respected for his *General Adaption Syndrome* theory, often referred to as GAS. Han's Selye was a professor at the University of Montreal and is best known for his work on stress and its relationship to physical and mental illnesses. He explains, the connection is not always clear. Selye has 33 books and 1600 scientific articles to his credit. He was the first one in 1938 to connect stress to illness. Hopefully, after reading the following, you will come to the same conclusion I did: stress plays a major factor in who gets sick and who doesn't. Even the distress of an impending illness can allow for disease to take hold. Stress is a *"dis-ease"* in itself. We must learn how stress affects our health and how controlling it will increase our chance of survival.

Cortisol is one of the body's stress hormones, and when elevated it can cause disease. If a person has high cortisol levels, their immune system's pH is usually on the acidic side.

> *"Researchers from around the world have slowly been uncovering the relationship between elevated cortisol levels and numerous chronic diseases."*
>
> Shawn Talbott Ph.D.

Having acidic pH in the body is bad, because an acidic pH is virus friendly. The body becomes acidic during stress, because the body's fight or flight mechanism is switched on. The fight or flight mechanism (of which the adrenal glands are a part) causes the body to dump sugar into the blood stream. The elevated blood sugar was intended to give us the energy required to run from or fight an attacker, *"fight or flight."* Our body's reaction to stress was meant to be a life saver. However, today when we are stressed from things, other than physical harm, sugar is left idle in the blood stream. Our body must struggle to keep the blood at an acceptable pH. This causes our body to pull calcium from other areas, such as our veins and bones, to keep our blood at a constant alkaline pH. The idle blood sugar results in chemical harm to the body, such as diabetes, cancer, arthritis, or susceptibility to illness and disease.

Think about it, if you were to pour acid on a table what would happen? It would burn a hole, right? Acid in the body is just as destructive to our tissues. If we don't run from an attacker, the idle sugar makes our body acidic. Our veins and organs are slowly compromised by the acidic condition. Cell walls become weakened and thin from being exposed to the acidic condition. When the cell walls are thin it is easier for viruses to penetrate and take advantage of our cell's RNA to reproduce. Viruses, bacteria and cancer thrive in an acidic environment. On the other hand, an alkaline environment inhibits the reproduction of viruses, bacteria and cancer. An alkaline environment keeps the cell membranes from being compromised by a virus. The stronger the cell membranes the harder it is for a virus to penetrate the cell and multiply.

I saw first hand how stress can affect disease when my mother passed, causing my cancerous tumor to more than double (you can read more about how stress affected my cancer in my book *A Journey Through Cancer.)*

I believe Dr. Hans Selye, the guru of stress, said it best when he was asked how he came up with his theory on stress and disease before becoming a doctor, while working in his clinical medicine introduction class:

> *"Since these were my first patients," Selye writes, "I was still capable of looking at them without being biased by current medical thought."*
>
> Gerald Gabriel, Hans Selye, pg 2

> *"Albert Einstein reportedly once said that his own major scientific talent was his ability to look at an enormous number of experiments and journal articles, select the very few that were both correct and important, ignore the rest and build a theory on the right ones."*
>
> *(Pg 61, The Great Influenza)*

Like Dr. Selye, I am not biased by current medical thought and, like Einstein, I love to read and draw from studies already presented to develop a new theory. Not being a doctor, I can look at things differently by putting pieces together that once were not connected. Also, I don't have to follow any preset rules when developing a theory. I am a researcher and use my research to look at problems in a different light.

Like Dr. Selye, I looked at the 1918 Bird Flu without the preconceived bias of a virologist, but as mathematics major, researching the information of those who went before me, the doctors, scientists and writers, concluding that stress was a significant factor in the reason why so many young people with good immune systems died in 1918. Managing stress will be a significant factor if or when the Bird Flu returns.

Max Von Pettenkofer, the second scientist, was a German trained doctor. In 1885 he was coming up with his own theory about how illnesses are acquired and passed on from human to human. He developed his theory at the same time as a rival and another German trained doctor, Robert Koch, was developing his own germ theory. Pettenkofer believed that more than one thing causes illness, whereas Koch believed only a germ caused illness. Pettenkofer thought that the chemistry or a combination of microorganisms resulted in illness. His theory was one of about four that were being debated at the time. Koch's theory has become the accepted theory by the medical community today. I will go into more detail of Koch's work in relationship to Pettenkofer in the coming pages.

Who is Richard E. Shope? He is a scientist, under the guidance of Paul A. Lewis, working at The Rockefeller Institute's animal pathology laboratory at Princeton. He came up with a theory in the1930's, while studying Swine Flu in pigs. He speculated the cause for the flu of 1918. He believed that Spanish flu (another name for the Bird Flu of 1918), like the Swine Flu was a combination of ailments that resulted in the Flu becoming deadly. He felt Swine Flu was caused by the combination of ( virus + swine lungworm + winter = Swine Flu ). He tried to prove his theory by using healthy pigs, infecting them with lungworm and the swine flu virus, then pouring ice cold water on them (to simulate winter). This he hoped would result in the pig obtaining Swine Flu. It worked with great results. Shope tried to further surmise that the Flu of 1918 was caused by a combination of factors: ( virus + Pfeiffer's bacillus + winter = 1918 flu. ) He was in essence trying to prove Pettenkofer's theory from 1885 that illness is caused by a combination of factors, not just a single pathogen. He was taking Pettenkofer's theory one step further, looking for the combination of substances that would result in disease. Shope also theorized that viruses could lie dormant, like the herpes simplex virus. This he felt explained why during June and July the 1918 flu cases were at all time lows.

If we look at Dr. Selye's work on stress and apply it to that time of year-- summer is a time of year when people are less stressed. The physical weather is better, more sunshine, less seasonal effectiveness disorders and more people are going on vacation. Less stress equals less disease. Also, viruses thrive better in drier weather, such as winter.

Back to Shope who believed that the virus would reappear when it was activated by some kind of stimulus (winter), it would trigger the virus to come back to life. This was a good explanation but the scientific community had some problems with his theory.

## SHOPES THEORY FAILED BECAUSE:

1. Many of those who died in 1918 had no signs of bacterial infection at all

2. In those that did have a bacterial infection, some had Pfeiffer's bacillus while others had staphylococcus or streptococcus.

3. Some cases were in August, not quite a winter month.

The contradictions in his theory did not totally discredit him but raised questions. In Crosby's book, he writes on page 303, *"Shope's theory is like Thomist philosophy or dialectical materialism: it may be wrong but it does provide plausible answers for the questions asked most often and does make comprehensible sense."* However, Shope's theory was correct. It is just that his assumption about his data was wrong.

Many other scientists tried to prove their theories for the 1918 flu but found that their experiments would work sometimes and not others, thus leaving them stumped. Shope was the only one that had a theory that could be reproduced. There is a reason for this, the other scientists could not reproduce their theories, because they used healthy animals and since healthy appearing animals do not always get sick, this would account for the inability to reproduce their experiments. Their animals also may not have experienced stress. Shope was the only scientist that introduced a stress into the equation. Stress is a big factor in disease ( virus + stress = disease ). Shope made a great discovery when he decided to use pigs in his experiment. Ask any pig farmer and you will find that pigs are naturally highly stressed animals. This is probably why Shope's pigs got Swine Flu, they were under stress. Shope made a mistake when he came up with the equation ( virus + lungworm + winter = Swine Flu ). If he had come up with the same conclusion that I did, ( virus + stresses = disease ) he would have made more sense of his data. The cold water acted as a stress factor for the pigs, not as a simulation of wintertime. This stress factor is the stimulus that Shope was looking for, and mentions in his work, when he said, *"Some kind of stimulus triggers the virus to come to life."* If he had tried his experiment eliminating the lungworms but used a stress factor for the pigs, his theory may have held up, regardless of what type of stress he chose.

All through Crosby's and Kolata's books scientist were coming up with plausible reasons for the flu, but they had trouble reproducing the results. Gina Kolata wrote a book, *"The Story of the Great Influenza Pandemic of 1918 and the Search for the Virus That Caused It."* I have found her information quite helpful. She explained how the scientist's had trouble in reproducing their experiments. I feel their trouble may have resided in the fact that they were using healthy animals or humans to perform their trials. Healthy humans should not get sick. They should have tried stressing out the animals or humans, then using their same technique; their results could have been different.

A human trial example of such an incident was the Deer Island Experiment, where M. J. Rosenau and Lieutenant Junior Grade J. Keegan obtained nine volunteers, trying to understand the transmission of the disease from human to human. The problem with their experiment was that the men (human guinea pigs) in their experiment were imprisoned sailors from a navel training center. They were free of stress, since they were not headed off to war. The men were not over exercising, nor staying out all night, and were also told that they would be granted their freedom for their participation in the trial, which could have actually made them happy. These imprisoned men were breathed on by sick people. They were subject to throat and nose swabbings from sick victims, and many other things. To Rosenau's surprise none of the men got sick. He went on to think his experiment was a failure. However, his experiment ends up showing us, if someone has no real impending stress and is given good news, such as an offer of freedom, they don't get sick. Basically, healthy people should not get sick.

If Rosenau and Keegan had used troops that were about to embark on their journey across the Atlantic to WWI, who had stayed up all night, drinking and smoking, their test results may have been different.

Instead they ended up proving that healthy people, given a positive outlook, will not get a disease. Several other scientists when trying their own experiments also ran into inconsistencies. Sometimes the animals got sick and other times they didn't. Stress could have caused the experiments to fail or succeed. If the animals were stressed it worked; if they weren't stressed, it didn't.

Robert Koch (Pettenkofer's rival) a German bacteriologist in 1884 laid down the rules by which suspect microorganisms were to be evaluated. Even though his germ theory is still accepted today as fact and has a lot of merit, it is missing two key elements: stress and the body chemistry environment. Stress by Selye's and Shope's information is a key missing factor.

The other missing factor is the body's chemistry. Remember when Koch was coming up with his theory, there was another rival theory on the horizons by Pettenkofer. Both Koch and Pettenkofer were German scientists trying to convince the world that their theory of the causation of disease was correct. John Barry writes in The Great Influenza about Pettenkofer, *"He insisted that Koch's bacteria was only one of many factors in the causation of cholera."*

Pettenkofer, wanting to prove his theory, decided to drink down pure cholera bacteria and had some of his students do the same. No one died and only two of his students got a minor illness. However, Pettenkofer's theory went on to be discredited when two cities in Germany, Hamburg and Altona, had an out break of cholera. One city, Altona, following Koch's advice, immediately began filtering their water, while Hamburg did not, following Pettenkofer's advice. Altona escaped the disease while Hamburg was ravaged. The problem with Pettenkofer's theory was that he did not know what the other causation factors were. He knew there was more to illness than one pathogen, but he hadn't found the other pieces to his puzzle yet.

Morton Walker, in his book, *Elements of Danger,* discusses cavitations at great lengths. Cavitations are bacteria pockets in the mouth. Bacteria we know can cause problems but its byproduct should be considered too. While the bacteria are in the mouth, it produces a byproduct toxin, which is even more deadly than the bacteria alone. Weston Price, a scientist, studied bacteria and its byproducts. In one of Price's studies he isolated the bacteria, putting just the bacteria into one rabbit and then putting just the byproduct toxin into another rabbit. The rabbit with the byproduct toxin died sooner than the rabbit with just the bacteria. This shows that the bacteria in the body in conjunction with its byproduct will cause a more serious disease then the bacteria alone. As the bacteria produces more waste the illness will become greater. Focusing only on the bacteria and not addressing the byproduct is like missing part of the equation. Price in essence proved Pettenkofer's theory that a combination of factors causes disease and death.

Koch was not completely wrong. Pettenkofer was not completely right. They both had a lot to contribute to the pathogen definition. Neither theory was exactly right on its own. To ignore the infecting agent, because your body's chemistry is healthy, is like saying, *"Since I am healthy I should be able to make it past a row of opposing football players."* Not a wise thing to do, since football players can be quite aggressive. Bird Flu is aggressive too. We should take every precaution possible to ensure we survive, like wear a mask to prevent infection. Even if you have the perfect immune system, you will still want to wear a mask, meditate, and exercise during the pandemic. A constant assault on your immune system will weaken your body's defenses. It will be up to you to keep your immune system strong.

Just as Pettenkofer should have cleaned up the water to prevent cholera outbreak, in conjunction with trying to find the other factors causing the disease. If we just use Koch's germ theory, then we can do very little to avoid becoming victims of the Bird Flu, other than trying to prevent exposure. If we understand the whole process of illness, that other things, besides exposure, can play a role in our health, then we can do a lot to get our immune system ready for an invasion.

## KOCH'S RULES TO IDENTIFY SUSPICIOUS PATHOGENS SUMMARIZED:

1. Microorganisms must be found in all cases.

2. Microorganisms must be able to be cultured outside the body.

3. The culture must produce disease when transmitted to healthy animals, which is identical to the original disease.

4. Microorganisms can be retrieved from experimental animals.

Rule three should contain a Selye Stress Factor (GAS) and a Pettenkofer combination factor which if corrected, number three, would read:

3. The culture and its' byproduct, when transmitted to a healthy but stimulated (stressed) animal must produce disease identical to the original disease.

This change in bacteriology is necessary for us to understand that if a pathogen has the ability to multiply, it will therefore have the ability to produce more byproduct toxins, and the more ill that person will become. A change in Koch's rules would have made some of the other scientists' experiments show positive results and made their experiments reproducible. If the other scientists only used the bacteria and not the organism byproduct, or if the animal was not stressed, both of these missing factors would cause a result to be inconsistently reproducible. Not knowing whether or not an animal was stressed in the experiments alone would render the experiment findings useless and difficult to collaborate. If the experiment contained only the filtered microorganism without its byproduct, this could change the experiment's results, because the animal's immune system may have been able to kill the organism before the organism could create a byproduct. The animal then may or may not show any symptoms.

In summary, Hans Selye, Richard Shope, Robert Koch and Max Von Pettenkofer are scientists whom have done a great deal of studying in their particular fields.

## IN SUMMARY

1. **Hans Selye** – Stress leads to illness
2. **Max Von Pettenkofer** – Combination of factors causes disease.
3. **Richard Shope** – Proved ( virus + stress = disease. )
4. **Robert Koch** – Exposure to disease can cause illness.

If you put their works together, collectively, it would explain why the 1918 flu became so deadly. They proved the theory, *"the pandemic of 1918 became deadly, because the virus was combined with several stresses."* Unfortunately, Pettenkofer had already died before 1900. Selye and Shope were both working during the 1930's independently, on different parts of the continent, unaware of each other's research and theories. If they had only met, the 1918 flu mystery may have been solved back then.

By using Shope's, Selye's, Koch and Pettenkofer's studies putting the conclusions together, we can understand the flu of 1918. Shope was trying to prove his own theory and was unable to obtain the explanations he was seeking. Selye's work, if applied to Shope's theory would have sent Shope's data results in a whole different direction. If Shope and Selye could have defined microorganisms differently, using Pettenkofer and Koch's theories, that too would have changed the summation of their data.

Now combining Shope, Selye, Koch and Pettenkofer's work to explain the Bird Flu, it was not the simulation of winter in Shope's experiment that was a deciding factor but the stress (Selye's stress factor) put on the pigs. It was also the combination of factors: exposure to the virus, the body's pH (Pettenkofer), not a single pathogen that promoted the illness. If Shope had attempted to simulate stress instead of winter, his theory would have held up.

# Appendix B

# Natural Air Purification System

Natural Air is a company that has developed air purifiers that have both ozone production and ionization. Their product produces ozone. Ozone is one of the most effective ways to clean and purify air. With their machines, overdosing on ozone should not be a worry, as long as the unit is used in accordance with the company's suggestions and is functioning properly. The Natural Air machines when tested only created a concentration of .03 ppm of ozone in a typical room. The average safe outdoor ozone level is between .05 ppm to .08 ppm. Since the concentration of the air in a room with the machine, is less than what is found outside, this should lessen your concern. The machines only restore the indoor air quality to what is found in outdoor air.

Natural Air puts out a tested product which produces ozone and both positive & negative ions. If a product only produces ozone and not positive & negative ions the EPA has shown that *"a room could develop unsafe levels of ozone."* If a machine produces ions in conjunction with producing ozone, the possibility of unsafe levels of ozone being produced is greatly reduced, because the ions are combining with particles, making them too heavy to stay in the air, causing them to fall to the ground, resulting in cleaner air. If you have only an ionizing machine, then you are missing the extra oxygen that is a byproduct of ozone. Remember, viruses do not do well in an oxygenated environment. Also, since ozone reacts with things that are not solid, without ozone you are losing this function of purification.

Why is ozone important in an air purifier? Ozone, as O3, will release an oxygen atom when combining with foreign gases in the air and the ions will combine with them, making them too heavy to stay airborne and knock them to the ground.

A lot of negative hype exists about the ozone producing machines. People are in fear of overdosing on ozone. The EPA tested some air quality ozone models by placing them on high (not the machines manufactured recommended settings) and found that the indoor Ozone levels came to be at unsafe levels.

Note, the machines were not used in accordance with the manufacturer's instructions. There was no documentation to indicate that the EPA studied to see if ozone was still dangerous, if the machines were used according to the manufacturer's instructions. In addition, I could not find any further information on what models they tested or if the models they tested only produced ozone and did not contain an ionizer in conjunction with the Ozone production.

Air purification machines with an ionizer could prevent a room from reaching the unsafe levels of Ozone found in the EPA study, because the ionizer would be taking the ozone out of the air, hindering the room from reaching toxic levels. Their study appears to be incomplete and misleading. If you are afraid of ozone, you may still want to obtain a machine, just in case you run out of masks.

We do not know if air purification machines will totally disinfect something like a mask from the Bird Flu, but it sure beats doing nothing and not being prepared.

## Appendix C

# City Guide For Preparing For The Bird Flu

Once the Bird Flu hits the US, a city should take notice, even if it is not transferable from human to human at that time, because once human to human transmission takes place there may not be enough time to set the needed procedures in place. First, a city should devise a Bird Flu Committee (BFC). The committee could include a city mayor, to five down: Maintenance Manager, Funeral Director or Medical Examiner, Hospital Director, frig or freezer business owner, Police and Fire Rescue Personnel, a neighborhood watch leader, building supply store manager, Vo-Tech or high school shop teacher. These people need to be identified by name. Cities will need to consider how certain companies should be compensated for the use of their facilities and expertise. This should be negotiated now when the threat is not pressing; to wait will hold up much needed preparations. The BFC needs to have a meeting to discuss a tentative plan of action in advance. Once the Bird Flu makes its way to being transmitted from human to human, the plan needs to be reevaluated. The plan should include a timeline and implementation procedures.

By far the best thing a city can do to prepare is to have enough body bags on hand for at least seven percent of their population. Most of the problems in 1918 stemmed from not having them. If you have body bags there will be less body fluid leakage. Less contamination will make people more willing to haul the bodies from the home to a gravesite. Remember, in 1918, bodies were found everywhere. At least with a body bag, they will be contained.

As soon as the flu has made the jump to human to human transmission the city will need to start organizing the city further, even if the human to human transmission is across the country. In a matter of days or weeks it could be knocking on your city's door. The more prepared the better your city will be.

At first the hospitals will not be overrun, and most deaths will occur there, but once the hospitals are filled to capacity a second phase of body processing will be required since people will begin to die at home. How will bodies be picked up? Who will do the job of picking up bodies? The city should count on needing far more city employees than they think should be required. Some of the employees will take ill and be unable to perform their duties. The city should also develop a form (see Bird Flu Death in the Household –What to do?) to be filled out when a family member dies, as well as a body cataloging system, prior to the first citizen taking ill. If the city staff is getting sick at the same time as everyone else, there will not be time to figure out what to do. This needs to be done well ahead of time. How will a family member let the city know someone has passed and is in need of pickup? How should the family prepare a body to transport for burial?

Each city needs a plan of action. San Francisco did not heed the warning of the east coast cities and was caught off guard in 1918. Many of the Cities and hospitals were running with fifty percent of their normal workers at the peek of the pandemic. Even though all fifty percent did not die, many people still came down with the flu at the same time and were unable to work. Our fair cities can do a lot to prepare for the flu.

How will the police protect us in the midst of crisis? The police should halt the sale of firearms as soon as a threat of a pandemic is realized. We do not want panicked untrained people owning firearms just prior or during a pandemic. Most people who own firearms prior to a pandemic usually have at least some fire arm training. Panicked people and guns do not mix.

The succession of leaders is necessary to assure the city will have leadership during a pandemic. As leaders fall ill there will be one to take their place. Knowing the next in line to head up the city will keep the city running. All leaders should be well informed about the cities comprehensive plan. The city then should start scouting out a place that could hold a mass graveyard. The graveyard should be able to hold approximately 7-10 percent of the cities population. It may be necessary for larger cities to have several different sites. The BFC should think about how it will organize and label each grave, and also how it will get the bodies buried. Pine boxes will be needed in several sizes. Who will make them? Where could the city store bodies waiting to be processed for burial? Is cremation a possible option? All of these questions need an answer. They should be answered now rather than later.

## CITY PLAN OUTLINE

1. Develop leadership at least five down from the mayor

2. Create a Bird Flu Committee

3. Develop a contingency plan

    A. Develop body identification procedure
        1) Hospital
        2) Citizens

    B. Body transportation to the gravesite
        1) Lawn maintenance trailers
        2) Sanitation vehicles
        3) School buses

    C. Body holding site
        1) Business with frig or freezer capacity

    D. Coffins
        1) Find a local place to set up shop
        2) Building supply store
        3) Vo-Tech school
        4) Have templates made for different body sizes

    E. Location for mass graves
        1) Plan for graves (labeling and recording)
        2) Assign grave diggers

3) When digging shall commence

F. Community outreach program

1) Notify citizens via:
   - Radio
   - Newspaper
   - Flyers
2) Designate who will inform them:
   - Police
   - Fire
   - Neighborhood watch leaders
3) Decide when, how and if you should hand out body bags

G. Maintain Order

1) Organize Street leaders
2) Police presence at medical sites, grocery stores, building supply stores and drug stores
3) Temporarily halt the sale of firearms.

Cities should take the time to prepare. In turn, citizens will feel comfortable knowing there is a plan and their city is watching out for them. They will know what is expected of them and what to expect from the city. This will dispel fear in the time of distress.

# Appendix D

# Hospital Preparedness Guide

In this section I will be talking about what doctors may want to think about in order to prepare for the Bird Flu. I am not trying to tell doctors what to do, but please consider this section when preparing for the Bird Flu. Doctors should address their attention to patients that the Bird Flu will affect most. Patients with respiratory problems, blood clotting problems, constipation, dehydration or other conditions that cause an acidic environment in the body are at high risk. Doctors may suggest that patients obtain a 6-month supply of medication.

If patients are taking drug blood thinners, doctors might want to replace them with a more readily available natural supplement, like capsicum or garlic (See resource section in the back of the book for natural supplement companies). It may be necessary to use natural, more available means during a time of pandemic. The more traditional drug sources may not be available and a natural product may be the only choice possible during a pandemic. Doctors, in the time of an infrastructure breakdown could be helpful to their patients if they have some knowledge of complimentary medicine. Patients should be given instructions on how to wean themselves off medication, otherwise they may go off cold turkey and cause more harm to themselves.

Our diet as a country will need to change. Doctors should warn their patients about mucus causing foods, such as dairy products, and encourage an alkalizing diet. Raw, whole foods, such as fruits and vegetables are very alkalizing and should be consumed during a pandemic. Sugars, white flour, white rice, candies, cakes, ice cream should be avoided. Meat consumption is very acidic and should be reduced until the threat of a pandemic is over.

Patients need to be counseled on the proper use of cough suppressants. If cough suppressants are used right away, they may hinder the body from expelling excess fluid from the lungs. Alternatives such as mullein and cherry bark are known for their mucus reducing ability.

Hospitals should have a plan for disinfecting a doctor or nurse before they return home. Even if a doctor or nurse is disinfected at the hospital, medical staff may want to also take a shower when they return home, making sure to use an apple cider vinegar rinse before toweling off.

Don't! Hospitals, please don't, over work your medical personnel!!!!! Yes, people may die, because doctors or nurses went home to get much deserved rest. Think of it this way, how many more will die if no doctors or nurses are well enough, or alive, to help save the sick and dying. They can be our heroes, but let's have them be responsible ones. Make sure the hospital has a plan to ensure that its doctors, nurses and staff stay healthy.

Hospitals should be set up to run on half staff, since many of their employees could be succumbing to the illness at the same time. As soon as the virus makes the jump to human to human transmission, the hospitals need to be on full alert. All elective surgeries should be reduced and then cut out altogether when the pandemic is in full swing.

Hospitals should start training *under staff* and cross training people who can fill in to work when the current staff is diminished. *Under staff* are people without medical education that will work during the pandemic. Many schools and businesses will be closed and those employees will need work during a pandemic. They can be trained to be in *under staff* positions ahead of time. They could do support work for the hospital, such as making beds, tagging bodies, making meals for patients and staff, etc. *Under staff* positions are emergency personnel for the hospital. They can receive money for their work and be guaranteed employment during a pandemic, provided they are not ill themselves.

## HOSPITAL PLAN

1. Emergency Staff scheduling, with half the employees out sick.

2. Medications needed to fight the flu.

3. Citizen notification plan - when to bring ill people into the hospital. (Radio or newspaper)

4. Admission Policy, so that the most ill people are admitted first.

5. Bedding capacity for 2% of the city population.

6. Alternate Hospital site
   A. Citizen Notification of alternate site: sign at the front door or out at the street
   B. College or high school Gym

7. Determine how many hours staff can work before mandatory medical rest is required

8. Develop a plan to disinfect doctors and nurses off premises before they return home to their loved ones.

# Appendix E

# Storage Formulas

The *"Usage Formula"* can be used to determine how much of a product you use in one week. This is necessary to determine how much of a product is needed to have in stock. The *"Usage Formula"* is not necessary for things like tampons, toilet paper, razor blades, or diapers; it is used for things like shampoo, juice, cereal, or milk.

## Usage Formula

**(Total amount of units in the product) multiplied by (fraction used) = amt of product used in one week**

**1/8** bottle of a **16 oz** bottle      **16(1/8) = 2** ounces used

## Determine how much you need for 6 months

Now you are going to use the information above. and multiply it by 4.2 to get your usage for one month and then multiply that answer by 6 to get how much you need for six months. The month factor we are using is just over four since there are usually more than four weeks in most months. This gives us our month factor = 4.2

## Need Formula

**(Amount used) (Month factor)(Number of months) = (How much is needed)**

## EXAMPLE FOR TOILET PAPER:

**2.5** rolls (**4.2**) (**6**) = **63** rolls of toilet paper needed for 6 months

Now comes the tricky part. If you buy toilet paper in 24 roll packages, how many packages do you need?

### Package formula is:

**(How much you need) divided by (how much comes in a package)**

So for toilet paper you would need to have in stock:

**63 / 24 = 2.625 packages**

That would mean three twenty- four roll packages on hand. Always round up. This means you will have extra, because if you round down you may fall short of your needs.

## EXAMPLE FOR SHAMPOO

Remember the answer from the usage formula:

**1/8** bottle of a **16oz** bottle **16 / 8 = 2** ounces

Now apply that to the need formula and we get:

**2(4.2)(6) = 50.4 ounces**

If 16 ounces come in a bottle, how many bottles do I need? The answer is found by using the package formula:

**50.4 / 16 = 3.15** bottles

This tells you for six month you will want to have 4 bottles of shampoo in stock, which will be more than enough for six months.

## IN SUMMARY WE NEED TO:

1. **Determine how much you use by using the Usage Formula:**
   **(Total amt of units in the product) multiplied by (fraction used) = amt of product used**

2. **Determine your need using the Need Formula:**
   **(Amount used) (Month factor)(Number of months) = (How much is needed)**

3. **Determine how many packages you need by using the Package Formula:**
   **(How much you need) divided by (how much comes in a package)**

4. **Purchase and store the amount of packages needed in step three. Continue to use and replace items to keep them as fresh and clean as possible.**

This formula can also be used to determine how much is needed for one to two years or more. The key is to find out how much you use and create a stock of what you use. Things that are not used or show little signs of being used, like mustard, should tell you to just have one or two extra on hand. By dating the box or bottle, over time you will see how much mustard you use in six months.

# Resources

## AIR AND WATER PURIFIERS

http://www.escapethebirdflu.com
P.O. Box 10111
Titusville, FL 32783

## SUPPLEMENTS

http://www.escapethebirdflu.com
P.O. Box 10111
Titusville, FL 32783
Supplements, herbs, essential oils

http://www.herbsforkids.com
1-800-232-4005
Liquid herbs for kids

http://www.boironusa.com
1-800-264-7661
Oscillococcinum and other Homeopathic medicines

http://www.airbornehealth.com
1-800-590-9794
Herbal & vitamin supplement for colds and flu

http://www.naturessunshine.com
1-800-453-1422
Essential oils, vitamins, herb combination, Target P14, PH Test Strips

http://www.qualityproducts.unfranchise.com
Powdered vitamins and supplements

## FOOD AND SEEDS

http://waltonfeed.com
1-800-847-0465
Grains, beans, dried milk, dried eggs, dried butter, dehydrated fruits and vegetables, Sprouting Seeds, Water Storage Supplies, Grinders, and Books

http://www.frontiercoop.com
1-800-669-3275
Herbs, spices, essential oils, supplements, natural cleaners, personal items, sprouting seeds, Dehydrated Foods.

## MEDICAL, CLEANING AND PERSONAL SUPPLIES

http://www.allegromedical.com
1-800-861-3211
N95 Masks, gloves, antiseptics and other medical needs

http://www.seventhgeneration.com
Phone orders through Gaiam 1-800-869-3446
Natural cleaners, disposable menstrual pads and diapers

http://www.gladrags.com
1-800-799-4523
cloth sanitary pads

http://www.diaperjungle.com
P.O. Box 42383
Phoenix, AZ 85080
cloth diapers

## GARDENING SUPPLIES

http://www.squarefootgardening.com
1-877-828-1188
All New Square Foot Gardening
By Mel Bartholomew

http://www.seedsofchange.com
1-888-762-7333
Organic seeds for growing fruits and vegetables. Groceries online

## MISCELLANEOUS

www. Holisticdental.org
Holistic Dental Association

Marianne Williamson
Audio - *Morning and Evening Meditation*

Dr. Andrew Weil
Audio - *Breathing, The Master Key to Self Healing*

http://www.vitamix.com
1-800-848-2649
grain grinder / Blender

http://www.mylifeinabox.com
(559) 325-6679
"My Life In A Box. A Life Organizer"
Organizing important documents.

Red Cross Disaster Services & Emergency Assistance.
For disaster relief, contact your local Red Cross chapter.
http://www.redcross.org
American Red Cross National Headquarters
202-303-4498

http://www.alpinesauna.com
1-866-697-2862
Far Infared Sauna

# References


Appell, Thomas, Never Get Another Cold, Irvine, CA VDP Publishing, 2004.

Barefoot, Robert R., Reich, Carl, M.D., *The Calcium Factor*, pg. 43-125, Wickenburg, AZ, Deonna Enterprises Pub., 2002.

Barry, John M., *The Great Influenza: the epic story of the deadliest plague in history*, New York, Penguin Books, 2005.

Berczi, Istvan, Dr., *A Personal Reminiscence*, http://home.cc.umanitoba.ca/~berczii/pge2.html

Bernstein, Richard K., M.D., *Diabetes Solution*, Boston, MA, Little Brown and Company, 2003.

Billac, Pete, *The Silent Killers*. 2006 Swan Publishing

Boyum, A., Wiik, P., *The Effect of Strenuous Exercise, Calorie Deficiency and Sleep Deprivation on White Blood Cells, Plasma Immunoglobulins and Cytokines*, Scandinavian Journal of Immunology, Blackwell Publishing, Feb. 1996.

Casau, Armelle, *When Pigs Stress Out,* HealthWorld U.S. N.Y., Published: October 7, 2003. http://query.nytimes.com/gst/fullpage.html?sec=health&res=9E00E3DE103CF934A35753C1A9659C8B63

Clausing, Chris, *The Bird Flu, and Vitamin C*, Health Keepers Magazine, vol. 8 issue, pg 10, and 11.

Crosby, Jr., Alfred W., *Epidemic, and Peace, 1918*, 1976 Greenwood Press, Westport, Connecticut

Crosby, Jr., Alfred W., *America's Forgotten Pandemic*, New York, Cambridge University Press, 1990.

Duffy, William, *Sugar Blues*, 1975, p. 121-135.

Dunne, Lavon J., *Nutrition Almanac third ed.*, pg. 246-247, New York, McGraw Hill, 1990.

Dyer, Wayne. W., Dr., *Official Website of Dr. Wayne W. Dyer*, www.drwaynedyer.com.

Forbes leadership Library, *Thoughts on Opportunity*, Triump Books, Chicago, 1998.

Gabriel, Gerald, *Hans Selye: the discovery of stress,* Scientific Learning, http://www.brainconnection.com/topics/?main=fa/selye.

Goodman, Sandra, Ph.D., *Vitamin C, The Master Nutrient*, chapter 6-13, http://www.positivehealth.com/permit/Articles/Nutrition/vitc13.htm

Gore, Al, An *Inconvenient Truth*, 2006.

Jarvis, D.C. M.D., Folk Medicine, Fawcett Crest Book, Greenwich, Connecticut, 1958.

Jensen, Bernard, Anderson, Mark *Empty Harvest*, p.76, 125-128, Avery Publishing Group, Garden City Park, New York, 1990.

Kolata, Gina, *Flu: The Story of the Great Influenza Pandemic of 1918, and the Search for the Virus That Caused It,* New York, Farrar, Straus, and Giroux, 1999.

Long, Laurie Ecklund, *My Life in a Box*, Fresno California, AGL Publishing, 2006.

Maier, Steven F., Laudenslager, Mark, *Stress and Health Exploring the Links*, Psychology Today, August, 1985.

Porter, Katherine Anne, *Pale Horse Pale Rider*: three short novels, NY, Harcourt, Brace & Company, 1939.

Quillin, Patrick, Ph.D., *Beating Cancer with Nutrition*, pg. 75-79,180,234-235, Tulsa, OK, 1994.

## References


Ritchason, Jack, *The Little Herb Encyclopedia*, Woodland Publishing, Inc, 1994.

Ritchason, Jack, *The Vitamin, and Health Encyclopedia Revised*, Woodland Publishing, Inc., 1996.

Selye, Hans, M.D., *The Stress of Life*, pg. Xi, 369-425, New York, McGraw Hill Book Co., 1956.

Shefferman, Mary R., *Stress Reduction - Part 1 of 3*, Modern Ferret

News, issue #28, August, 2002. http://www.ferretnews.com/issues/modern-ferret-news-28.html

Siegel, Bernie S., M.D., *Love, Medicine and Miracles*, New York, Harper & Row Publishing, 1986.

Stauth, *David, Vitamin E Loss Through Smoking Increases Health Risks*, Oregon State University, OSU News & Communication Services, Vitamin E Loss Through Smoking Increases Health Risks, 4/14/05, http://oregonstate.edu/dept/ncs/newsarch/2005/Apr05/smoking.htm

Tenney, Louise, *Todays Healthy Eating*, pg. 40, 50, Woodland Publishing, Inc., 1986.

Walker, Morton, D.P.M., *Elements of Danger*, Charlottesville, VA, Hampton Roads Publishing, 2000.

Weil, Andrew, M.D., *Is Stress Making You Fat?* http://drweil.com/drw/u/id/QAA323853, 1/16/2004.

*"There is no security
on this earth,
only opportunity."*

Douglas Macarthur

# Index

## Index

# What You **Must Do**

# to

# Escape

# the

# Bird Flu

If you are interested in purchasing any of the products talked about in **What You Must Do to Escape the Bird Flu** such as an air purifier, humidifier, personal air purification system or supplements they can be ordered through our website at:

**www.escapethebirdflu.com**

# The Storage System

The storage system is a CD and Workbook that is designed to help you determine your storage needs.

## WORKBOOK AND CD

- **What you should store**
- **How much to store**
- **When to replace your storage food**
- **Where to buy items for storage**
- **Storage food recipes**

The kit includes charts and worksheets for you to develop your own storage plan. The plan will save you money by telling you when and how you should rotate your stock. Don't let your precious storage spoil, learn when to eat it and when to replace it!

# Other Books
## *by*
## *Brendanne Phillips*

## *A Journey Through Cancer*

***"A Journey Through Cancer"*** is the story of one woman's dramatic and emotional journey through breast cancer. This story not only ends with a cure but a long awaited miraculous birth of a child. Brendanne Phillips' journey is different from most cancer stories because it is the story of a young woman who chooses not to follow the conventional means of treatment. The courage and strength needed to follow this path while raising two small children is both motivating and encouraging. ***A Journey Through Cancer*** will appeal not only to those women who want to treat cancer using conventional and alternative methods, but also to that growing number of women raising small children while dealing with this illness.

Brendanne grew up with her mother battling breast cancer. She saw first hand how cancer can affect people. This book is not a recipe on how to heal cancer but an inspirational story on how one woman beat the odds. Her story will offer hope and inspiration to others finding themselves in the same position.

To order *A Journey Through Cancer* from any book store use the ISBN number 1-4137-1708-X. Or use the order form found in the back of this book.

# Immune System Coach

Along with her books Brendanne is an Immune System Coach, offering information and one-on-one consultations:

- ★ **Locating what your immune system is lacking**
- ★ **How to change your diet and your family's diet**
- ★ **Help in getting fussy children to eat healthy**
- ★ **Educating your spouse**
- ★ **Exercising tips**
- ★ **Questions to ask your Doctor**
- ★ **Supplement training; finding the best ones for you**
- ★ **What books you should be reading**
- ★ **How to deal with stress**
- ★ **How to find a doctor that will work with you**

If you are interested in learning more about this life changing program, you can contact Brendanne by

Email at: bren@escapethebirdflu.com

Or by snail mail

Brendanne Phillips
P.O. Box 10111
Titusville, Florida 32783

# About the Author

## *Brendanne C. Phillips, B.S.*

Cancer survivor and health educator, Brendanne Phillips is no stranger to working with a life threatening illness. She was diagnosed with breast cancer in 1998. Using many techniques unknown to the medical community, her cancer was kept under control until the cause was discovered. Through thorough research and the help of many doctors, Brendanne was able to uncover the cause of her cancer.

Brendanne's interest in research into health and healing began in 1995 when her young daughter began having ear infections. Brendanne started reading and discovering uncommon medical techniques that helped her daughter. She now understands there is more to health than we realize. Using these uncommon medical techniques Brendanne saw her daughter's full recovery within one month.

In 1998, she was challenged with her own development of cancer. Her mother and her mother's three sisters all had developed breast cancer, so it was no surprise when Brendanne received the same diagnosis at the young age of 35. She put her research abilities to the test once again, reading everything she could find on cancer. This proved to be a success when, after two years of research, she was able to discover the cause of her cancer that would then produce a cure.

At the first indications of a Bird Flu probability, she began her research efforts, a third time. Again, using researched information she developed a family plan in the event the Bird Flu should arrive. After researching for over a year and a half, she was disappointed by the information being given out to the general public. Knowing there is more we can do in our everyday lives to prepare for the Bird Flu, she continued her research and decided to put her research into an easy to read book: *What You Must do to Escape the Bird Flu* for everyone to benefit.

*"A Loving heart*
*is the beginning*
*of all knowledge."*

Thomas Carlyle

# Quick Order Form

Brendanne Phillips
P.O. Box 10111
Titusville, FL 32783
Email orders to: bren@escapethebirdflu.com

| | | |
|---|---|---|
| *What You Must Do to Escape the Bird Flu* | $19.95 | ________ |
| *A Journey Through Cancer* | $19.95 | ________ |
| *Storage System* | $199.99 | ________ |

Subtotal __________

Shipping __________

Tax (Fla. Res.) __________

**Total** $____________

**Shipping:** $3.00 (U.S.) for the first book and $2.00 for each additional book.
**Canada:** $5.00 for the first book and $3.00 for each additional book
**Sales tax:** Please include 6% sales tax for products shipped to Florida addresses
**Payment:** ___ Check ___ Credit Card ___ Visa ___ MasterCard

Card #: ________________________________ Exp. date: __________

Name on card: ______________________________________________

Address: __________________________________________________

City: ________________________ State ______ Zip _______________

Telephone: (____) ___________________________________________

Email ______________________________________________________

❑ Please send FREE! Bird Flu updates to my email address.